SAVAGE WILL

ALSO BY TIMOTHY M. GAY

Assignment to Hell:
The War Against Germany with Correspondents Walter Cronkite,
Andy Rooney, A. J. Liebling, Homer Bigart, and Hal Boyle

SAVAGE WILL

WILL

THE DARING ESCAPE OF AMERICANS TRAPPED BEHIND NAZI LINES

Timothy M. Gay

NAL
CALIBER

NAL Caliber
Published by the Penguin Group
Penguin Group (USA), 375 Hudson Street,
New York, New York 10014, USA

USA | Canada | UK | Ireland | Australia | New Zealand | India | South Africa | China

Penguin Books Ltd., Registered Offices: 80 Strand, London WC2R 0RL, England
For more information about the Penguin Group visit penguin.com.

First published by NAL Caliber, an imprint of New American Library,
a division of Penguin Group (USA)

First Printing, September 2013

LIBRARY OF CONGRESS CATALOGING-IN-PUBLICATION DATA:

Gay, Timothy M.
Savage will: the daring escape of Americans trapped behind Nazi lines/Timothy M. Gay.
p. cm.
Includes bibliographical references and index.
ISBN 978-0-451-41913-2 (hardback)
1. World War, 1939–1945—Campaigns—Albania.   2. World War,
1939–1945—Campaigns—Mediterranean Region.
3. Medical personnel—United States—History—20th century.   4. Nurses—United
States—History—20th century.   5. Combat survival—History—20th
century.   6. Escapes—Albania—History—20th century.
7. Rescues—Albania—History—20th century.
8. World War, 1939–1945—Secret service.   I. Title.
D766.7.A4G39 2013
940.54'21965—dc23   2013015549

Printed in the United States of America
1   3   5   7   9   10   8   6   4   2

Set in New Caledonia
Designed by Sabrina Bowers

PUBLISHER'S NOTE
While the author has made every effort to provide accurate telephone numbers and Internet addresses at the time of publication, neither the publisher nor the author assumes any responsibility for errors, or for changes that occur after publication. Further, publisher does not have any control over and does not assume any responsibility for author or third-party Web sites or their content.

ALWAYS LEARNING   PEARSON

To the memory of my father-in-law, Judge Ellis A. Oualline, and to his late brothers, Judd and Royce, all of whom served with great distinction in the U.S. Army Air Forces during World War II.

I will summon every resource to prevent the triumph of death over life. . . . I will be untiring in the performance of my duties. . . . This I will do. I will not falter, in war or in peace.

—The sworn oath of USAAF flight evacuation nurses in World War II

Vdekje Fashizmit! Liri Popullit! ("Death to Fascism! Freedom to the People!")

—The sworn oath of Albania's Communist Partisans in World War II, accompanied by a clenched fist and a pound of the chest

Our bodies were dying, numb with the swift ebb of our strength; we had only a savage will somewhere inside that kept us going.

—Sergeant Lawrence Orville Abbott, describing how the trapped Americans eluded the Germans near Gjirokastër, Albania, on December 29, 1943

PRINCIPALS

THE NURSES

	HOMETOWN
Lt. Gertrude Dawson	Pittsburgh, Pennsylvania
Lt. Agnes Jensen	Stanwood, Michigan
Lt. Pauleen Kanable	Richland Center, Wisconsin
Lt. Ann Kospco	Hammond, Louisiana
Lt. Wilma Lytle	Butler, Kentucky
Lt. Ann Maness	Paris, Texas
Lt. Ann Markowitz	Chicago, Illinois
Lt. Lois Watson McKenzie	Oak Lawn, Illinois
Lt. Frances Nelson	Princeton, West Virginia
Lt. Helen Porter	Hanksville, Utah
Lt. Jean Rutkowski	Detroit, Michigan
Lt. Elna Schwant	Winner, South Dakota
Lt. Lillian Tacina	Hamtramck, Michigan

THE MEDICS

	HOMETOWN
Sgt. Lawrence O. Abbott	Newaygo, Michigan
Sgt. Charles Adams	Niles, Michigan
Sgt. Paul Allen	Greenville, Kentucky
Sgt. Robert Cranson	Sandy Creek, New York
Sgt. Jim Cruise	Brockton, Massachusetts
Sgt. Raymond Eberg	Steelville, Illinois
Sgt. William Eldridge	Eldridge, Kentucky
Sgt. Harold Hayes	Indianola, Iowa
Cpl. Gilbert Hornsby	Manchester, Kentucky
Sgt. Gordon MacKinnon	Los Angeles, California
Sgt. Bob Owen	Walden, New York
Sgt. John "J.P." Wolf	Milwaukee, Wisconsin
Sgt. Charles Zeiber	Reading, Pennsylvania

THE AIRMEN

Lt. Jim Baggs
Sgt. Richard Lebo
Sgt. Willis Shumway
Lt. Charles "C.B." Thrasher

HOMETOWN

Savannah, Georgia
Halifax, Pennsylvania
Tempe, Arizona
Daytona, Florida

THE ALBANIAN RESCUERS

Hasan Jina
Kostig Steffa
"Pandee"
Rahman Runi
Tare Shyti
Quani "Johnny" Sigeca

HOMETOWN

Elbasan region
Berat
Elbasan region
Elbasan region
Tragjas, Vlorë
Berat region

BRITISH SPECIAL OPERATIONS EXECUTIVE OPERATIVES

Maj. Philip Leake
Maj. C. Alan Palmer
Maj. Anthony Quayle
Maj. H. W. "Bill" Tilman
Capt. Victor Smith
Capt. Jon Naar
Lt. Gavan B. "Garry" Duffy
Sgt. H. J. "Blondie" Bell
Cpl. Willie Williamson

HOMETOWN

Dulwich, South London
Reading, Berkshire
Southport, Lancashire
Wallasey, Cheshire
Merseyside, Lancashire
Hendon, Northwest London
Leeds, Yorkshire
Islington, North London
Leith, Scotland

U.S. OFFICE OF STRATEGIC SERVICES OPERATIVES

Army Maj. Lloyd G. Smith
Army Maj. S. S. Kendall
(a.k.a. Dale McAdoo)
Army Maj. Harry Fultz
Marine Lt. John Hamilton
(a.k.a. Sterling Hayden)
Marine Sgt. Nick R. Cooky

HOMETOWN

State College, Pennsylvania
Hornell, New York

Salem, Indiana
Upper Montclair, New Jersey

Dilles Bottom, Ohio

CONTENTS

CONTENTS

MAPS

SAVAGE
WILL

SAVING THE "FLOWER OF AMERICAN WOMANHOOD"

Screened by a covey of destroyers, the U.S.S. Iowa slipped away from Senegal under a veil of secrecy. It was unusual for an American battleship to be trolling Africa's Atlantic waters that far south. But the *Iowa* was no ordinary battlewagon. For much of the past month, she had been carrying the world's most powerful human being. Her proud crew had even installed a special circular bathtub to accommodate the disabled commander in chief.

Allied naval officials were petrified that Nazi spies had spotted President Franklin Delano Roosevelt that Thursday afternoon, December 9, 1943, as he inspected Free French troops in Dakar. An FDR sighting, the brass feared, would be instantly relayed to the Berlin headquarters of the Abwehr, Adolf Hitler's spy agency, which in turn would flag the *Unterseeboot* (U-boat) captains preying in the Atlantic. The president's battleship, sure to be steaming west, would make for fat pickings; if torpedoed and sunk, it would also make for a staggering Nazi propaganda coup. Roosevelt's convoy was on high alert as, sonar pinging, it zigged and zagged toward the Americas.

FDR had just completed three weeks of grueling diplomacy, a furtive sojourn via ocean armada, transport plane, flying boat, and motorcade that had taken him past Gibraltar to Oran, Tunis, Cairo, Teheran, and back to Cairo again. After Allied troop morale-building stops in Tunisia, Malta, Sicily, and Senegal, he was finally heading back home aboard the *Iowa*.

Roosevelt was ground down from his travails. At three different Middle East summit meetings, he was compelled to play both mediator and referee, juggling the oft-clashing aims of America's British, Russian, and Chinese allies, not to mention the territorial ambitions of prospective ally Turkey. Forced to coddle the prickly personalities of British prime minister Winston Churchill, Soviet premier Joseph Stalin, Chinese generalissimo Chiang Kai-shek, and Turkish president İsmet İnönü, the president had earned some rest and relaxation. Sailing the high seas, a favorite pastime from his days as assistant secretary of the Navy, was the perfect tonic. FDR spent much of the next week lounging on the *Iowa's* deck, basking in the December sun under a crumpled fedora.

As he sunbathed, the president could not have been happy with the reports he was getting about how the Anglo-American offensive in Italy had slowed to a crawl. Two full years after the U.S. entered the war, and thirteen months after launching their joint Mediterranean campaign, British Tommies and American G.I.'s were caught in a stalemate against Hitler's Wehrmacht.

Almost as frustrating for FDR, the Brits and the Americans were also struggling to gain traction on a top-secret rescue operation that preoccupied his heart and mind. Four and a half weeks earlier, an American cargo plane carrying twenty-six medical professionals, half of them female nurses, had crash-landed in Nazi-occupied Albania. The resilient young Americans were still trapped behind enemy lines. Roosevelt was incensed. In his mind, the Allies' clandestine action agencies, the British Special Operations Executive (SOE) and the U.S. Office of Strategic Services (OSS), seemed paralyzed. FDR fancied himself a devotee of the dark art of espionage; he even had a "mole" at SOE's Mediterranean headquarters slipping him inside dope on the Brits' rescue efforts. America's chief executive was fed up with what he viewed as foot-dragging.

Roosevelt couldn't do much about breaching the enemy Gustav Line in Italy's Apennine Mountains. But, by God, he could do something about getting those poor nurses out of Albania!

By Sunday evening, December 12, the ship's-position log put the *Iowa* convoy in midocean, at N38.5 latitude and W44.0 longitude, roughly halfway between the archipelago of the Azores and Bermuda. It was two and a half hours into cocktail time when Roosevelt reached for his telephone.

Jon Naar, a twenty-three-year-old captain from the Hendon borough of northwest London, was alone on duty at SOE's headquarters at the Rustum Buildings in Cairo. He was working late, recording the latest "gen" (SOE slang for intelligence) from the British liaison officers (BLOs) secreted in the southern Balkans. His phone rang at 2330, a half hour before midnight.

"Captain Naar here," he answered, in his brisk British public school way.

The connection was remarkably free of static. A female operator said, "Please hold for the president."

A moment later, there was no mistaking the patrician Yankee accent, so famous from radio broadcasts and movie newsreels.

"This is Franklin Roosevelt," the voice growled. "Why the fuck is it taking you so long to get those nurses out?!"

Seven decades later, the ninety-three-year-old Naar recalled the surreal moment.

"Before I could explain the logistical complexities of trying to extricate thirty Americans in the dead of winter from a mountainous country occupied by three divisions of the Wehrmacht and several brigades of pro-Nazi Albanian collaborators entirely in control of all the major roads and airfields, the president said, 'Captain, if any one of those girls is so much as *touched*, there'll be serious consequences!'"

After a slight pause, FDR snapped, "They are the flower of American womanhood. They must be saved at all cost!"

Naar heard a loud click. His conversation with the leader of the free world had ended as abruptly as it had begun. The entire exchange had lasted less than thirty seconds.

Receiver in hand, Naar sat at his desk, trying to make sense of what had just transpired. He'd had no warning that America's pissed-off president would be calling. Naar always prided himself on giving straight answers to straight questions, yet he'd barely managed to get in a word edgewise.

He had been given no opportunity to inform President Roosevelt that a BLO was, at that precise moment, risking his life trying to lead the Americans back to freedom. Or that SOE's operation in Albania had been turned upside down because of the stranded nurses and medics.

The hour was so late that there was no one at SOE headquarters to whom Naar could recount his presidential butt-chewing. But first thing the next morning, the young officer briefed his boss, Major Philip Leake, head of B8, the Albanian section of SOM, Special Operations Mediterranean.

Leake, the peacetime headmaster of south London's elite Dulwich Prep, was seething. "That's typical of the Yanks!" he snarled.

"Throwing their bloody weight around with absolutely no clue of what's really happening!"

Naar and Leake knew the truth about the Albanian rescue effort—or at least thought they did. But from the moment Allied intelligence was first alerted about the marooned Americans, the entire episode had been shrouded in fog.

CHAPTER 1

LOST IN THE FOG OF WAR

Straining their eyes through the clouds, second lieutenants Lois Watson McKenzie and Agnes Jensen stared, disbelieving, as antiaircraft artillery tracers tore perilously close to their medical transport. The dank mist that enveloped the plane made the reddish slugs seem even more malignant. Sitting several rows behind the nurses, Sergeant Lawrence Orville Abbott, a medic and a car buff, likened the ack-ack tracers to sparks from a coughing engine.

Ugly black bursts soon erupted off both wings, rocking the plane. The fog was so dense it was as if the deadly fusillade were being fired from some unseen netherworld.

One minute their Dakota C-53 was lowering its wheels and swooping toward the ground, eliciting cheers from the twenty-six nurses and medics on board. The next moment they were gasping for air as the plane aborted its landing. Seconds later they were slammed against their seatbacks as the transport lurched skyward.

And now somebody was shooting at them! An ominous *clang!* began rattling from the tail section.

But who was doing the shooting? And why?

Since leaving Sicily four hours earlier on what should have been a routine hop to southern Italy, they'd been flying blind, lost in the dismal November slop for what seemed an eternity, desperately seeking terra firma and a place to land. They'd finally spotted a coastline and, a few minutes after that, an airdrome, only to discover that it was controlled by someone hostile.

Was it the Axis enemy? Had they somehow wandered over that part of Italy still dominated by the Germans?

As it climbed, the plane began to twist and turn, first one way, then the other. Clearly the pilots were taking evasive action, scrambling to hide in thicker cloud cover. The frenetic swerving could mean only one thing: Hostile fighter planes were now chasing them!

McKenzie, Jensen, Abbott, and company tried to remember their training and not succumb to panic. Jensen glanced across the aisle and saw a nineteen-year-old male medic "shaking like a leaf." Before long, through a break in the clouds, they glimpsed craggy white mountaintops. They knew their fuel couldn't last much longer.

These young Americans were—quite literally—trapped in the fog of war. Most of them would stay trapped for the next sixty-two days, unwittingly dragging into the mire the president of the United States, two Allied special ops agencies, the British Balkan Air Force, the 12th and 15th U.S. Army Air Forces, the USAAF's public relations command, and hundreds of flinty Albanian Partisans. The operation to rescue the Americans became so obtrusive, in fact, that SOE officers worried it was undermining their efforts to help the Albanian resistance eradicate the Germans.

Before the ordeal finally ended, it would ensnare two future movie stars, one English and one American; one of the most decorated soldiers in English history; the British Empire's most renowned explorer and mountaineer; the scion of Britain's largest cookie fortune; and the Cold War's most notorious traitor. To spring the final group of Americans, Allied special operatives and their Albanian cohorts would concoct a subterfuge so audacious that it rivaled the Central Intelligence Agency's *Argo* rescue in Iran thirty-six years later.

Fog is so pervasive throughout the classic film *Casablanca* that it's practically a member of the cast. Released in the fall of 1942, the movie was still new to the British troops hunkered down in Italy a year later. When the Tommies at one camp watched the climactic scene when Humphrey Bogart's character, Rick Blaine, guns down the reptilian German major Heinrich Strasser (Conrad Veidt) on a murky airport tarmac, the Brits hollered, almost in unison: "Stretcher bearer!"

Too many Allied stretchers were needed in the Italian campaign—and there weren't enough medics and nurses to bear them. Italy was, as the great American war correspondent Ernie Pyle wrote, a "tough old gut." Its forbidding terrain lent itself to the diabolical warfare at which German Army Group C commander *Generalfeldmarschall* Albert Kesselring had become expert.

Kesselring had convinced Adolf Hitler in the fall of 1943 to let him use Italy's mountains to wage a defensive brawl. He directed his men to detonate roads and bridges, fall back to high ground, turn and fight, then slip away to blow up more roads while retreating to even higher ground.

For Allied soldiers, it amounted to a nonstop artillery barrage launched from one thorny summit after another. The Germans' Volturno Line gave way to the Bernhardt Line, which gave way to the Gustav Line, and so on, as the Allies slogged through increasingly miserable winter weather.

The Italian campaign was a morass, but it was also a moving testament to the coalition of nations that rose up to stop Nazi Germany. Allied ground forces may have been called the "U.S. Fifth Army" and the "British Eighth Army," but they included Canadians, Brazilians, Frenchmen, Poles, Czechs, New Zealanders, Australians, Indians, Free French Moroccans, Palestinian Jews, and others.

Certain habits and uniforms may have seemed peculiar to American eyes. But the international soldiers fought with great tenacity and spilled blood in the same troubling amounts.

The reason so many air evacuation nurses and medics were summoned to Bari, Italy, in early November 1943 was that General Bernard Montgomery's British Eighth Army had just launched an offensive across the River Trigno. On November 3, the 11th Infantry Brigade—Tommies from East Surrey, Lancashire, and Northamptonshire, plus a battalion of men from the famed "Ox and Bucks," the Oxford and Buckinghamshire Light Infantry—combined with three Royal Tank units from the 4th British Armoured to capture a rugged ridge outside San Salvo. Four days later, with the Ox and Bucks and Indian infantry near the point, the Eighth pushed the Germans out of the village of Paglietta and off Mount Calvo south of the River Sangro.

As always, Italy's high ground had been seized at catastrophic cost. Every day, scores of wounded men were shipped to Bari and Grottaglie, 150 miles to Monty's rear. As the casualties piled up, so did the calls to Catania and other air evacuation bases in the

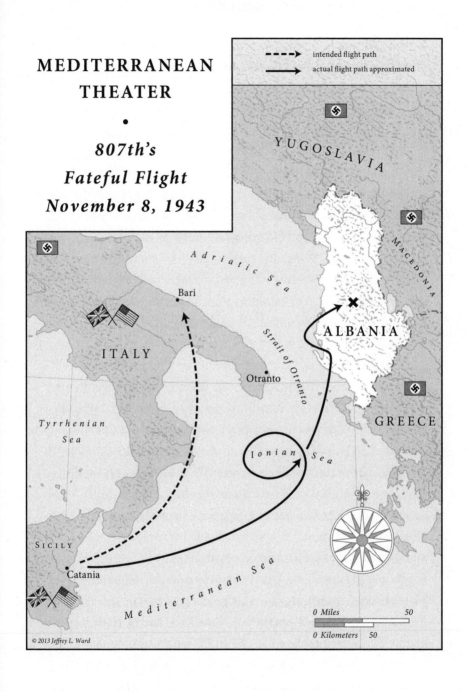

MEDITERRANEAN
THEATER

•

807th's
Fateful Flight
November 8, 1943

intended flight path
actual flight path approximated

YUGOSLAVIA

MACEDONIA

Adriatic Sea

Bari

ITALY

ALBANIA

Strait of Otranto

Otranto

GREECE

*Tyrrhenian
Sea*

Ionian Sea

SICILY

Catania

Mediterranean Sea

0 Miles   50

0 Kilometers   50

© 2013 Jeffrey L. Ward

Mediterranean. The Eighth Army needed more stretchers, more morphine, more sulfa powder, more nurses, more medics, and more evacuation planes. And it needed them right away.

At the moment the C-53 lost its bearings, SOE lieutenant Gavan Bernard "Garry" Duffy, a demolition expert trained by the Royal Engineers, was somewhere in central Albania, teaching Partisan guerrillas how to blow up roads, bridges, and the occasional Nazi staff car. The SOE had taught Duffy to operate underground, right under the nose of the enemy. Established in part to help downed Allied airmen elude capture, Duffy's cloak-and-dagger outfit went by the portentous moniker "Middle East Operations and Escapes."

The Yorkshireman, an émigré from Dublin, was obsessed with weaponry, spare with small talk, not exactly a prototypical ladies' man. But he was twenty-four years old, fiercely competitive, proud of his ability to survive in harrowing conditions, single, and human.

When SOE's headquarters in Cairo, transmitting through bulky B2 wireless sets, informed the BLOs scattered around Albania that a plane full of American nurses had gone missing, Duffy was determined to win the race to rescue them. He hustled toward SOE's southern Albanian mission, hoping it would give him a leg up in finding the distaff Americans. It did.

Helping coordinate Duffy's movements in Albania was his SOE comrade in Cairo, the officer fated to become the object of FDR's telephone ire, Captain Jon Naar. Like Duffy, Naar was one of the younger members of the SOE team, but the Londoner brought an entirely different skill set to special ops. He was a wordsmith, adept at solving the *Times* of London's inscrutable crossword puzzle in a matter of minutes, fluent in German and French, and competent in Russian and Arabic. As B8's intelligence officer, he was responsible for keeping Leake and the BLOs in the field apprised of the rapidly changing positions of enemy and friendly forces in Albania. He devised a top-secret map for Leake and others in the "need to know." Plotting the course of the crash-landed American party became his major preoccupation in the late fall and winter of 1943–1944.

Naar spent hours every day updating his elaborate map, trying to figure how the BLOs could carry out their primary mission to make themselves a "bloody nuisance" to the occupying Nazis without being seriously diverted by the rescue of the Yanks. With Lieutenant Duffy trekking toward SOE's mountain hideout, Naar began moving his "Duffy" stickpin south and east.

The SOE captain also kept tabs on Albania's resistance leaders. That fall, a Partisan commander with a handlebar mustache and a thirst for Axis blood named Hasan Jina was bushwhacking Nazis and their collaborators in central Albania. A few miles south in the town of Berat, a multilingual school superintendent and father of five named Kostig Steffa, who doubled as a Partisan brigade commander, was nervously eyeing enemy troop movements. Meanwhile, an admirer of American democracy named Tare Shyti, who distrusted Communists almost as much as he detested Fascists, was shuttling between the inland capital of Tirana and his home along the Adriatic coast near Vlorë. As he traveled, the father of four and savvy prewar business executive took careful note of how Wehrmacht and collaborationist sentries examined his papers.

That November, OSS captain Lloyd Smith was in Bari, Italy, the very place that the C-53 was supposed to have landed. Smith, a native of State College, Pennsylvania, looked like the Penn State varsity wrestler he had been a few years before. Thick necked and squat shouldered, he was built like a fireplug. Smith, too, had been taught to torment the Germans through sabotage. Soon the twenty-four-year-old would be tasked with scaling Balkan hills to bring thirty trapped countrymen home from behind enemy lines.

It was the height of irony: To get the marooned Americans out through the underground, Duffy, his SOE comrades, Smith, and a flock of gritty Albanians had to sneak them across some of the highest ground in Eastern Europe. To pry the Americans out of the Balkans, Allied operatives resorted to tactics that transcended cultural boundaries: cutthroat threats and gold-sovereign-fueled bribery.

There's a reason "byzantine" and "balkanized" are part of our lexicon. The former means mysteriously complicated; the latter, hopelessly divided. In the winter of 1943–1944, those young Americans and the brave people seeking to rescue them would be besieged by both.

CHAPTER 2

FURTUNA OVER THE IONIAN

A *rough storm in the seas that surround Italy is so* dreaded that the word for it—*furtuna*—doubles as a Latinate lament for bad luck. It's the obverse of Fortuna, the mythological Roman goddess of good fortune to whom centuries of legionnaires prayed on the eve of battle.

At dawn on Monday, November 8, 1943, as thirteen female nurses and twelve male surgical technicians with the 807th Medical Air Evacuation Squadron (MAES) readied themselves to fly from Sicily to the Italian mainland to tend to wounded British comrades, *furtuna* was about to foist itself on them. A squall then off the Neapolitan coast was churning south by southeast, on a vicious collision course with anything in its path. The tempest turned out to contain as much geopolitical intrigue and recrimination as it did ice and sleet.

The young people in the 807th were a microcosm of 1940s America. Most were small-town kids from places like Indianola, Iowa, and Winner, South Dakota. But there was a smattering of city-bred twenty-somethings, too. They were the children of farmers, factory hands, mill workers, secretaries, lumberjacks, railroaders, and housewives.

Most of their surnames—Abbott, Lytle, Nelson, Adams, Porter, Hayes—smacked of Middle America and Main Street: They sound like characters in a Sinclair Lewis novel. But some were of ethnic extraction, too: a Rutkowski, a Markowitz, a Tacina. Whether WASP or immigrant, farm boy or city girl, they were about to get to know one another—and themselves—far better than they ever intended.

No training, no matter how intense, could adequately prepare America's young people for the cataclysm of world war. That was especially true for the nurses and medics of the 807th MAES, all of whom had received at least some measure of survival training. But no classroom lecture could teach them how to withstand frostbite or beat back pneumonia and unrelenting dysentery. No obstacle course could condition them to hike up a mountain amid a howling blizzard, or elude a firefight between rival guerrilla bands, or conceal themselves in the bush to avert a Nazi patrol.

Until they joined the service, most had never strayed far from home. Four thousand miles removed from the nearest soda shop, *furtuna* was about to wallop them in ways their worst nightmares could never have imagined.

Sicily's weather in early November 1943 mirrored the Italian mainland's: It was dreadful. Members of the 807th had gotten word late on Friday, November 5, that several of them would be flying from their base at Catania to Bari, Italy, the next morning to pick up ailing soldiers from the British Eighth Army. But the fog and rain were so bad that the flight was scrubbed on the sixth and again on the seventh. Since a big offensive had been launched along the British front, casualties were climbing—and so was the Brits' tension about getting their men cared for.

As the weekend wore on, more members of the 807th were added to the Bari mission. At 0730 Sunday morning, a cluster of them had actually climbed into a transport plane before the flight was called off. By that evening, roughly a third of the 807th's eighty-odd-person contingent of nurses and medics was committed to flying to Bari as soon as the weather cleared.

Monday morning, November 8, brought a slight break. The forecast predicted that the icy storm then hitting Italy's Tyrrhenian coast a couple hundred miles north would not arrive over the route to Bari until midday. There was enough time, officials reckoned, to make the quick 260-mile jump over the Ionian before the bad weather hit.

At that point, members of the 807th had been in Catania for more than a month. Most had been on missions to Bari, where a massive Allied hospital complex was then taking root. The nurses and medics by now knew the drill: They'd fly to the Bari airfield, where they'd be met by trucks and ambulances carrying wounded soldiers and on-the-ground medical personnel. There they'd review individual charts, get briefed by field physicians, nurses, and medics, pitch in to take care of emergencies, then supervise the transfer of injured soldiers onto special medical transport planes.

They enjoyed visiting Bari. The deserting Germans had left behind a bawdy nightclub next to the airstrip. Once their eyes adjusted to the darkness, the Americans realized the place featured etchings of nude women.

Since there was a possibility that they'd be spending the night in Bari with perhaps a little social time at the club if things didn't get too crazed, each tossed a change of clothes, some toiletries, and maybe a pack or two of cigarettes into the musette bags they liked to sling over their shoulders.

Although their Catania quarters were cramped, the 807th's female officers weren't exactly roughing it: Most were bunking in *villas marittima* that had survived the depredations of war. The modest bungalows were tucked onto a terraced hillside on a cobblestone *strada* not far from the sea.

Noncommissioned officers in the 807th didn't have it quite as soft. Most of the medics were jammed with privates and corporals in hastily thrown-together huts.

That morning, the nurses slipped on Army Air Force–issued slacks, which they'd learned were not only warmer but more functional than skirts. Most of them, fortuitously, also grabbed marine-blue trench coats with woolen liners; their names had been stenciled on the coat front. Not so fortuitously, most put on AAF oxfords instead of boots. Since it was raining, they also wore galoshes over their shoes. The galoshes kept their shoes drier but were hardly designed for hiking. Most of the nurses were wearing their light blue Army Nurse Corps dress caps with a narrow brim.

The medics, never imagining that they'd need anything heavier, donned slate-green field jackets meant for temperate weather. But at least most of them had put on boots with heavy socks. The men were proudly sporting their peaked flight hats with the AAF's gold-and-blue piping.

Sicily's sun had just peeked over the Ionian. Together with another medical outfit bound for the Grottaglie field hospital just south of Bari's, the 807th's delegation piled into jeeps. They were heading toward Catania Main Airfield, the little airdrome that, three months earlier, the Brits had spilled so much blood capturing.

Sandwiched between the southeastern slope of Mount Etna and the sea, halfway between Messina and Syracuse on Sicily's eastern shore, Catania had been devastated when Montgomery's XIII Corps ran into stiff resistance thrown up by Kesselring's 29th Panzer Grenadiers and other crack enemy troops. Much of the city's picturesque Roman-era antiquity had been reduced to rubble. It was in and around Catania in July and August of 1943, in fact, where Montgomery first exhibited the indecisiveness that would come to bedevil his American counterparts, not to mention many of his underlings.

Confusion and dithering also reigned at Catania Main the morning of November 8—as they often did at Allied airfields in the Mediterranean Theater of Operations (MTO). The base at that point consisted of little more than a dilapidated shack, a half-destroyed hangar, and a bumpy dirt runway that had been expanded to handle medium-weight bombers. AAF engineers and Sicilian laborers had been patching up the runway. Parked on the tarmac was a mixed batch of cargo transports, B-25 Mitchell bombers, the odd P-40, Piper Cubs, and other scout planes.

Even at that early hour, the place was packed: Too many servicepeople needed to get too many places that morning. There weren't enough planes to go around. No one was sure how the weather would affect flying conditions.

So the 807th's members cooled their heels, smoking and killing time. Some dug into their bags, pulling out books, magazines, and decks of cards.

Second Lieutenant Lois Watson McKenzie spotted a couple of B-25 bomber pilots from whom she'd hitched a ride a few days earlier. The bomber boys were heading to Bari, too, so McKenzie, a South Side Chicagoan never reticent about speaking her mind, asked whether members of the 807th could ride along. After a few minutes of spirited back-and-forth with the airbase command, McKenzie's request was denied. The brass's rationale was that the 807th had enough personnel to fill a transport; the entire outfit, therefore, had to wait until a cargo plane was available.

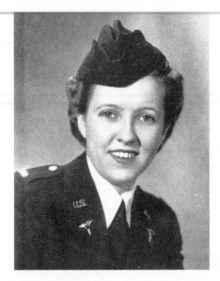

Second Lieutenant Lois Watson, March 1943.

The B-25 took off without them, but—in a portent that the base command should have heeded—ended up turning around and coming back; the weather was too dicey. Yet flights out of Catania continued that morning, even though the 12th and 15th U.S. Army Air Forces canceled virtually every bombing mission in the MTO that day.

By that point in the unit's history, members of the 807th had been around one another for close to half a year. They'd trained together at Bowman Field in Louisville and been squeezed into the same troopship across the Atlantic and through the Straits of Gibraltar. Friendship and, in certain cases, rivalry had been forged from nurse to nurse and medic to medic.

Yet most of the nurses didn't know the medics very well—and vice versa. Perhaps it wasn't all that surprising: The nurses were officers, the surgical technicians enlisted men. Fraternization wasn't just frowned upon; technically, it was forbidden. A few had gotten friendly working elbow-to-elbow in field hospitals and on medical transports, but for the most part they had stayed in separate orbits.

U.S. medical air evacuation had come a long way since being instituted in the 1920s to enhance the survival prospects of Marines wounded in the Nicaraguan bush while chasing anti-American guerrillas. Two decades later, as World War II deepened, AAF officials essentially made up a training regimen as they went along. Between 1942 and the end of 1944, some fifteen hundred nurses and nearly a thousand enlisted men graduated from special flight training. Eighteen medical air evacuation squadrons eventually were formed, each consisting of approximately twenty-five nurses, five doctors, one clerk, and sixty or seventy medical technicians.

By any standard, medical air services in World War II were a remarkable success. Of the more than a million Allied casualties evacuated by air, fewer than fifty died en route.

Before they got to Bowman in the spring and summer of 1943, the women and men in the 807th had been through various forms of military medical training. All had volunteered for air evacuation duty. Back then commercial airline stewardesses had to be nurses, so there was a natural synergy between the professions. About a third of the nurses in the 807th had been peacetime flight attendants.

The nurses were thrown right into the fray at Bowman. On day one, they were drawing blood from draftees waiting in line at Louisville General Hospital. On day two, they were teaching the medics how to extract blood and wrap bandages.

McKenzie remembered being handed a booklet on proper bandage techniques one evening and told she was teaching a class on it the next morning. She continued to lead coeducational instruction on bandaging, which caused much tittering as they got to various parts of the body.

"Flight Nurse school was grueling," McKenzie wrote five decades later. "Room inspections (dime bouncing on the bed), classes and afternoons of drill, calisthenics, hikes, survival swimming, etc. By [the] time you went to bed, you ached all over."

To get them used to flying in rough conditions, planes would take the trainees on long rides up and down the Ohio Valley, doing loop-the-loops. McKenzie steeled herself not to vomit by repeating a mantra: "I won't get airsick! I won't get airsick!" It worked.

But she was relieved when a fellow nurse did get nauseated; the pilots mercifully cut out the barrel-roll stuff and returned to Bowman.

The group, nurses included, had to learn to identify at quick sight Allied and enemy planes. They all had to master an obstacle course that included crawling under barbed wire stretched a scant foot and a half aboveground and ducking live ammunition. It was so exhausting on a broiling Kentucky afternoon that they'd finish a run and practically pass out.

Since they'd be transporting wounded soldiers by air, they learned to spot symptoms of oxygen deprivation, and what to do if an air mask at high altitude suddenly became inoperable. Lest they be forced to crash-land, they also learned how to navigate by compass and read maps with penlights.

Over time, they learned to work in teams of two, since in a combat zone, one medic and one nurse would be assigned to each evacuation plane. The same teaming approach was used to guide emergency room training at Louisville General.

All this intense preparation was the brainchild of the 807th's commander, redheaded Major William P. McKnight. Red McKnight drove the nurses and medics hard. But they grew to admire the boss with the strawberry mustache. Out of affection, they called him "the Old Man."

In late August of 1943, McKnight and the 807th got orders to travel by train to their North Atlantic embarkation center, Camp Kilmer, New Jersey. The nurses got twelve-hour passes, which they used to go sightseeing in New York City. Since they were clad in handsome military garb, everyone wanted to buy them drinks and meals. Two of the 807th's nurses were squired to the famed nightclub 21, where they whiled away the early morning hours, barely leaving themselves enough time to taxi back to the camp for the strict 0600 curfew.

After another day of waiting, they were taken to their portside departure point. With a military band serenading every step, they dragged their duffel bags aboard the transport SS *Santa Elena*. As the convoy pulled away from New York, everyone gathered on deck to admire the Statue of Liberty for as long as they could. Lieutenant Jean Rutkowski of Detroit couldn't help but think how tearful her Polish immigrant parents had been in 1907 when they glimpsed the statue on their way to Ellis Island. The *Santa Elena* was part of a sizable armada that, the nurses and medics learned in midvoyage, was heading toward the Mediterranean theater.

As noncoms, the medics were packed belowdecks, sleeping in hammocks. The nurses, as officers, had slightly roomier quarters; still, their cots were crammed end-to-end and side-to-side, with barely enough room between them to maneuver. Rutkowski and a couple of other nurses were relegated to the brig, which wasn't as stark as it sounds; the lockup at least had running suds. Each morning Jean and her friends filled a helmet with warm water so that some of the men could shave in comfort.

Their convoy steamed across the Atlantic, constantly drilling for a possible U-boat attack; they watched corvettes throw depth charges and the *Santa Elena* crew members readied themselves to abandon ship. Eventually, they negotiated Gibraltar, where the convoy split into two. The *Santa Elena*'s gaggle docked at Oran, Algieria. The 807th spent three nights in Oran before the *Santa Elena* and three other ships shoved off for Bizerte, Tunisia, arriving on September 6—five days after the British Eighth had attacked the Italian mainland at Reggio di Calabria, and three days before the U.S. Fifth would do the same at the Gulf of Salerno.

A British antiaircraft unit was planted across the road from the nurses' tents in Tunisia. The Brits, no doubt angling for social interaction, helped the women dig latrine trenches and foxholes and rigged up an outdoor shower. McKenzie remembered the nurses and their British friends swimming in the Bay of Bizerte and partying at a hole-in-the-wall they nicknamed "the Club."

But not everything was fun and games in Tunisia. On one of their first nights, as they enjoyed an outdoor movie, the Germans unleashed an air raid. With sirens wailing, they all scrambled toward the concrete bunkers that the Nazis had built before abandoning Tunisia the previous spring. Rutkowski followed a male British lieutenant into a bunker that was equipped with a cot, a table, two chairs, and a couple bottles of wine. She accepted his offer of a glass of wine, which helped calm her nerves. Everyone survived the raid.

Tunisia was only an interim home. As soon as living quarters were arranged in Catania, the 807th was transferred to Sicily. The nurses and medics were now part of an MTO medical operation that had already evacuated thirty-three thousand wounded Allied soldiers and prisoners of war from North Africa and Sicily—with many thousands more to come.

At some point after dawn on November 8, Gilbert Hornsby, a corporal with the 802nd MAES, a unit that had been in the MTO since American troops first stormed Moroccan beaches a year earlier, approached his counterparts in the 807th about hitching a ride to Bari. Six days before, Hornsby had somehow gotten separated from his outfit, which was operating out of the western half of Italy. The 802nd's mission was to evacuate injured G.I.s from the battleground of the U.S. Fifth; the 807th's job, meanwhile, was to concentrate on transporting wounded Tommies with the British Eighth on the peninsula's eastern side. Once on the ground in Italy, Hornsby figured he'd cadge a ride west.

The twenty-one-year-old youngster from Manchester, Kentucky, was told he could jump in with the 807th, but there still was no plane available. Hornsby tossed aside his large barracks bag and perched himself next to the rest of the gang. He had two cartons of cigarettes stowed away, which in the days to come would make him one popular corporal.

Finally, around 0745, the commander of the 52nd Troop Carrier Wing told the 807th members that a C-53 transport would be taking them to Bari. Most in the group didn't know it, but their C-53, per the wing's direction, would be flying to Italy that morning with two other transports in a three-plane formation.

The Dakota C-53 Skytrooper was a converted C-47, a military workhorse known pre- and postwar as a DC-3. C-47s and their wartime offspring differed from civilian DC-3s, but only slightly: Their floors were thickened, the better to absorb antiaircraft fire, and they were retrofitted with large doors, the better to handle sizable cargo.

More than ten thousand C-47s of various stripes were manufactured during the war. As Sergeant Orville Abbott of the 807th, who ended up owing his life to one, put it, "[C-47s] flew everybody and everything, from brass hats to paratroopers, and from tank parts to a crate of eggs." By the fall of 1943, C-47 supply planes had already been credited with helping turn the tide at Guadalcanal in the Pacific theater and proven indispensable in North Africa, Sicily, and Italy.

A C-53's innards, like those of its sister ship the C-54, had been ripped out to accommodate eighteen litters and various pieces of medical equipment, including a huge medicine chest. But the AAF had ingeniously designed the cabin so that stretchers could be attached by a series of clamps and brackets. For a flight to a combat zone, like the one the 807th was taking to Bari that morning, the litters could be detached to handle regular passengers. Bucket seats were then screwed into the floor and sides.

It was a sturdy ship but not a big one. A C-53 had two Pratt & Whitney engines and a wingspan of ninety-five feet, but ran just sixty-four and a half feet from nose to tail—only four feet longer than the distance from the pitcher's rubber to home plate. The Catania Main ground crew knew that exactly twenty-six bucket seats had to be set up for that plane's flight to Bari.

In misty rain, McKenzie and twelve other 807th nurses, all second lieutenants; Orville Abbott and eleven other 807th medics, all technical sergeants; and Gilbert Hornsby, the straggler corporal from the 802nd, lined up to climb aboard the C-53.

Abbott and a couple of other medics had gotten to know the copilot in Catania. He was a second lieutenant, a drawling, wise-cracking strawberry blond from Savannah, Georgia, named Jim Baggs. But no one in the 807th was acquainted with the main pilot, Lieutenant Charles "C.B." Thrasher from Daytona, Florida. Nor did they know the other crew members: the radio operator, Sergeant Dick Lebo from Halifax, Pennsylvania, or the crew chief, Sergeant Willis Shumway from Tempe, Arizona.

That morning's mission marked the first time that the four airmen had flown together—a fact that probably wasn't volunteered to the nurses and medics as they clambered aboard.

Maybe it was the lack of familiarity with one another, or being thrown into the mission at the last minute, but key items on the preflight checklist somehow got overlooked. No crew member, for example, thought to make sure there were enough parachutes and Mae West life preservers for everyone on board. The radio and compass most likely went untested. No one seemed to know that day's password command for air-to-ground radio transmission and

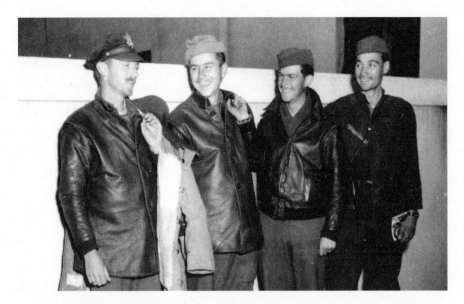

(Left to right) Second Lieutenant and copilot Jim Baggs, First Lieutenant and pilot C. B. Thrasher, Sergeant and radio operator Dick Lebo, Sergeant and crew chief Willis Shumway.

vice versa. They would be flying close to enemy lines in bad weather; yet the only firearm on board was a Thompson submachine gun with just thirty rounds of ammunition.

Second Lieutenant Agnes Jensen, a farm girl from western Michigan, was the first inside the plane. At the grand old age of twenty-eight, "Jens," as her pals called her, was one of the 807th's senior nurses. Per her usual custom, the veteran of three previous combat zone air evacuation missions threw her gear onto the right-hand-side window seat before settling into the seat next to it. The first bucket was uncomfortable because it was stuck next to the radio desk; a series of knobs and wires popped out at eye level.

C-53 bucket seats were made of metal and uncomfortably chilly. In the dank cold of a November morning at an altitude of eight thousand feet over the Ionian Sea, they weren't likely to get warmer.

Elna Schwant, a sassy brunette whose worldliness belied her

backwoods South Dakota upbringing, sat next to Jens. Schwant had a sardonic way about her that Jens found amusing. A few rows behind them, just inside the cargo door, sat another tart-tongued colleague, Lois Watson McKenzie.

Most of the nurses were situated behind Jens and Schwant on the right side, with the medics sitting opposite. Sergeant Paul Allen, at nineteen years old the youngest member of the squadron, male or female, sat across from Jensen and Schwant. A row behind Allen was Hornsby, the hanger-on, with Abbott just behind him. Across the aisle from Abbott was Pauleen J. "Paula" Kanable, a Wisconsin native whose gift for profanity would come to impress even the most hard-bitten of the noncoms.

Swearwords or no, after three days of sitting around, they were pretty much talked out. The books and magazines came back out; so did decks of cards, mostly for solitaire. A cross-aisle, cross-gender game of four-handed rummy broke out in the back.

One of the 807th's physicians, Captain Robert Simpson, had accompanied the group to the airfield. Simpson and pilot Thrasher conferred for a few moments at the head of the cabin. Then Simpson, a gregarious sort, stepped forward to address the group, confirming that there was indeed a cold front brewing but that it was not expected to hit the region until later in the day.

There should be plenty of time to get to Bari, Simpson said with a smile. Eyes twinkling, he facetiously inquired whether anyone had any "last words" they cared to share.

"Just spread the word—keep 'em flying!" someone bellowed from the back. Many of them were chuckling as they reached for their seat belts.

"Keep 'em flying," indeed. They weren't just watchwords of the U.S. Army Air Forces; the phrase could have been the motto of the Allies' entire Mediterranean campaign. Keep flying, keep fighting, keep pushing forward, no matter how bloody, no matter the cost.

Army Aircraft 42-68809 and its big white USAAF star went wheels-up at 0815. Despite bumpy winds, the takeoff was routine. So were the first few minutes of the flight.

Before long, however, the passengers couldn't help but notice that the puke-green sea was roiling; huge whitecaps were visible from several thousand feet. Angry black clouds inked the northwest sky. The big squall suddenly seemed much closer than several hours away.

Trying to keep their minds occupied, Agnes Jensen and Elna Schwant began chatting about the different places they wanted to explore in Italy once the Germans retreated. Ann Maness, their friend from Texas, who at that moment was sitting a couple of rows back, had just finished a special assignment in newly liberated Naples. Maness had taken advantage of a rare day off to visit the ruins of Pompeii, returning to Catania full of wide-eyed wonder.

Just then the C-53 got caught in a shear of wind so violent that Jens was amazed they came out of it right-side up. Had the passengers not been wearing seat belts, their heads would have bashed against the cabin ceiling. The plane seemed to groan with each flip of its wings. Anything that wasn't tied down, including their musette bags, began ricocheting around.

In a memoir written five decades later, Jens averred, "Nurses and medics had been trained too well to allow what they felt internally to be reflected on their faces. Fear and panic were contagious, and medical personnel were determined not to start or feed either."

The guys in the cockpit were not medical personnel; unbeknownst to the nurses and medics, the airmen were plenty panicked. First Lieutenant T. E. Yarbrough, the lead pilot in the three-plane formation, ordered the Thrasher-Baggs plane to stay on his right, or eastern wing, and to descend five hundred feet to seventy-five hundred feet. The other transport was told to fly on Yarbrough's left wing and ascend five hundred feet to eighty-five hundred feet. By fattening the distance among the planes, Yarbrough was hoping to reduce chances of a midair catastrophe.

But what Yarbrough didn't know was that Thrasher's radio was getting balky and soon—the crew later claimed—would be damaged by lightning. Yarbrough also didn't know that Thrasher and his men were having trouble with their compass. Just maintaining visual and radio contact with Yarbrough's lead plane proved untenable.

Radioman Lebo, looking increasingly aggravated, kept toying with the radio knobs next to Jensen and Schwant. Years later, once the odyssey's tortured blow-by-blow was pieced together, the nurses and medics learned that just twenty-five minutes into the flight Yarbrough spotted ice forming on his wings and directed the other pilots to activate their deicers.

Soon enough the cloud cover was so thick the passengers could not see the plane's wingtips—let alone any transports flying nearby. The temperature inside the C-53 was so bracing that Jens slipped a magazine between her rear end and the metal seat—and still found herself shivering.

Agnes Anna Jensen was a survivor. Life tested her when she was just a toddler—and never stopped. She somehow managed to keep the Grim Reaper at bay until her ninety-fifth year.

She was tall and lithe, with etched Scandinavian cheekbones, a regal nose, and mirthful green eyes that interviewers would later describe as "gunmetal" and "translucent." Her frame was slender and athletic, not unlike Katharine Hepburn's; she liked to wear her wavy brown hair in long curls that bobbed behind her ears.

Jens was born in December 1914, in Proctor, Minnesota, the sixth of ten children of Danish immigrants. Lauritz Jensen, a farmer, and his bride, Anna, had emigrated to the Minnesota prairie to find a better life. Agnes was barely out of the crib when her family was forced to flee the Moose Lake fire, one of the deadly conflagrations that ravaged the Upper Midwest. The

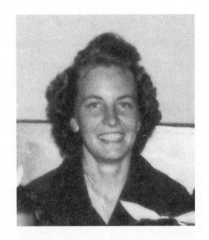

Agnes Jensen, 1944.

Jensens were among the thousands of farm families that lost virtually everything in the 1918 blaze. Hoping the area would prove less prone to natural disaster, Lauritz moved his brood to western Michigan, to the farming hamlet of Stanwood. Each young Jensen was expected to pitch in.

One of the many curiosities of the 807th's story is that its two furtive note takers and future memoirists, Lieutenant Jensen and Sergeant Lawrence Orville Abbott, were both western Michiganders. They grew up in adjoining counties no more than thirty miles apart. Yet they didn't know each other as kids and—despite the shared trauma they experienced as young adults—never became great friends.

Along with her siblings, young Agnes went to Stanwood's one-room schoolhouse through the eighth grade. She showed so much promise that her parents wanted her to continue her studies—but there wasn't a high school nearby. They arranged for Agnes to leave the farm and stay fifty miles away in Big Rapids, where she worked as a nanny so she could attend school.

After graduating from Big Rapids High in 1932, she moved cross-state to study nursing at the Henry Ford Hospital in Detroit. Unattached and eager to see the world, Jens and a friend talked each other into joining the Army nursing corps in February of 1941. They didn't give the potential of America being dragged into a global conflict a second thought.

Jens and her friend were training at Fort Benning, Georgia, when the news of Pearl Harbor hit, disrupting everyone's holiday plans. Her ten-day furlough was postponed twice before she was able to visit her family in Stanwood. Jens fibbed and assured her immigrant parents that an overseas nursing assignment would be no more dangerous than walking across a busy street. When she got back to Fort Benning, "They asked for volunteers for the Philippines, [with] signups right away," she recalled. "I was just sick I missed that. I didn't see the notice in time. [It would have been] ten thousand miles on somebody else's money."

It turned out that Jens still got her ten thousand miles' worth of excitement, but in a different theater of the war. She volunteered for flight evacuation in early 1943 and was sent to Bowman Field for special training. More experienced than most of the MAES nurses, she was entrusted with a leadership role.

Jens never informed her mom and dad that she had signed up for air evacuation duty. Planes made her folks nervous; they would have spent too much time fretting about her.

Lieutenant Jensen's unease didn't improve when she realized that the sheen she figured was another bank of fog was, in fact, the top of the sea. A few minutes before it felt like the plane was being forced skyward; now it was practically skimming along the waves. It dawned on Jens that she should have insisted on checking for life rafts and preservers. They weren't within easy reach; if forced to ditch, the passengers would be in trouble.

Lebo, annoyed, kept barging out to wrestle with the radio. At one point he left the door to the cockpit ajar. The passengers could see bewildered looks on the faces of the crew. It was not reassuring.

On and on they flew. Jensen, McKenzie, Abbott, and the rest hoped it wasn't in aimless circles—but it sure felt that way. As time dragged on, there was virtually no communication from the cockpit: "Nothing, nothing, nothing!" Jens would recall.

They'd been in the air for nearly two hours—already late for Bari, they reckoned.

Their log documented that Thrasher, despite the erratic radio, got through to the Bari tower two hours and sixteen minutes into the flight—at 1031. He asked them to provide a weather report. The Bari radio operators challenged the crew to share that day's password: They didn't know it. Bari broke off the transmission.

Nineteen minutes later, Thrasher tried again, this time requesting that the Bari tower activate its radio beacon to guide the plane to the airbase. Again, the operator demanded that Thrasher identify the password. When he couldn't, the request was denied.

Ten minutes later Thrasher attempted a third time; again he was rebuffed.

At 1135 Thrasher got through to the tower long enough to ask for a radio "fix"—but Bari lacked the proper equipment. At 1145, the Bari tower finally acceded to Thrasher's pleadings and turned on its beacon. But by 1155 the tower was no longer in contact with the plane. By noon the C-53 was truly flying blind.

The passengers knew none of this, of course. All they knew was that the cabin temperature had precipitously dropped. Jens slipped a second magazine under her derriere and resumed shivering.

Now it didn't seem like they were flying in circles. The clouds were beginning to break up; it felt like the plane was hewing to a straighter line. Not long after, Lois McKenzie saw a scary-looking waterspout that she swore was sucked up into the clouds like an apparition.

"Lois Watson, Oak Lawn, Illinois," which is how the just-married Lieutenant McKenzie was listed in the original missing-in-action press coverage, conjures a carefree upbringing in a leafy suburb, of flirting over chocolate malteds at the corner drugstore and dancing to swing music at the club Saturday night. Even the photograph of the uniformed nurse that the Chicago papers ran with the story—a sandy brunette with dimpled cheeks, a pug nose, and impish eyes—fed the image. Yet nothing could have been farther from the real adolescence of Lois Eileen Watson.

She never really resided in Oak Lawn; her parents moved there only after she left home to go to nursing school. Lois was, through and through, a Chicago kid. She grew up in Englewood, a dodgy stretch of the South Side where Al Capone and his capos called the shots in the twenties. Back then Englewood was made up of immigrants and working-class whites; it was full of loud hustlers and street urchins outrunning cops and truant officers. Lois was often at the head of the pack.

Her dad, Harry Dee Watson, was a near-lifelong railroader who'd grown up in Wyanet, not far from Rock Island. The youngest of four kids, he dropped out of school at the age of fourteen and two years later watched his mother die. He worked at a series of odd jobs until serving in the Great War. The November 1918 armistice took place just as Harry's outfit was being readied to go overseas.

After the war he worked for the Chicago Junction Railroad, then moved to Viola, Illinois, to take a job at a rendering plant. One day, still wearing grease-stained work clothes, he was walking a cow back to its pasture. In the field he spotted a pretty girl picking raspberries and struck up a conversation. Her name was Leila Mae Chesley; she was five years his senior and the youngest of eight children of a family far more prominent in Viola than the Watsons had been in Wyanet. When she first met Harry, Leila's Mae's heart was broken; her boyfriend had been killed during the war. Her parents, Willam T. Chesley and Ann Catherine Patterson Chesley, were blue blood cousins whose ancestors had emigrated from England in the seventeenth century. Her class-conscious father was unhappy that Leila Mae took up with a boy beneath her station, then became unhinged when she got pregnant without benefit of holy matrimony.

Leila Mae and Harry eloped and got an apartment on the South Side. Harry found work at the Illinois Central Railroad's Chicago Produce Terminal, eventually becoming switch foreman.

Harry was, in Lois's recollection, fun-loving and engaging, a raconteur who enjoyed teasing kids and blaring jazz tunes on a clarinet or a saxophone. He was a self-taught Renaissance man who enjoyed plumbing Chicago's museums and planetariums and was a mainstay at "A Century of Progress," the city's 1933–1934 World's Fair. He also wrote a geneaological history that traced his ancestors' migrations.

Lois always lamented that he never had the chance to go to college; with some formal education there was no telling what her old man could have accomplished. Harry liked to celebrate paydays by bringing home gifts for Lois and her younger (by seventeen months) "buvver"—little Lois couldn't pronounce "brother"—Wayne.

Leila could be dour; she kept her children in check by uncorking a facial sneer—a malicious expression that Lois, to her chagrin, apparently inherited.

Early on, Lois developed a rebellious streak that no maternal smirk could tame. The Watsons' mother-daughter clashes led to a rift that never quite healed. Harry's efforts at reining in his daughter tended to be halfhearted.

"I remember one incident when I was about sixteen years old," Lois wrote. "We were sitting around the supper table. The battery had been stolen out of our garaged car. Dad made the comment that it had to be someone I knew as I was the only one that knew that kind of people. With that, I threw my plate at him. He jumped

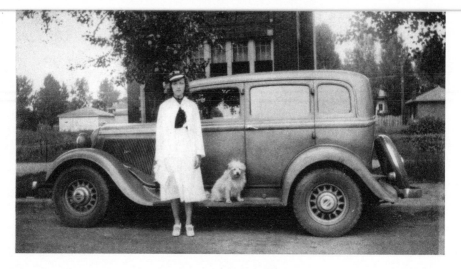

Lois as a teenager, 1938.

up and started chasing me down the hallway. He tripped and fell. We both laughed, thus ending the incident."

Lois never backed down when neighborhood toughs tried to bully her or her little brother. She once retaliated against an older girl who was taunting her "buvver" by dramatically pouncing on her from a tree; the fight turned so nasty, with threats and counterthreats of vengeance, that both sets of parents were forced to intervene.

She confided years later to her daughter Phyllis that a date once dropped her off well past curfew. Mr. Watson, agitated, was waiting on the apartment stoop. As the boyfriend's auto pulled up, her father barked, "Get inside right now, young lady!"

Lois never got out of the car and told the boy to gun the accelerator. She stayed out all night, making her parents heartsick.

Her sophomore year she was so reckless that her frequent absences got her thrown out of Parker High. Thanks to a kindly "adjustment teacher," the school relented and allowed her to reenroll. But she stayed defiantly lippy. Her senior year she carried three marijuana cigarettes in her purse. She never smoked them, but liked to brandish them for effect.

On the evening of June 16, 1938, when Lois received her diploma at the Chicago Civic Opera House, Parker High's female principal handed her the sheepskin, eyed her up and down, and jabbed, "Well, I'm certainly glad to see *you* go." To which Lois rejoined, "Not half as glad as I am to be getting out of this hellhole."

The battles with her parents had only started. Against the Watsons' wishes, Lois became engaged to a young man. But she broke things off in theatrical fashion, chucking the engagement ring out the apartment window. Neighbors thought a prowler was stalking the block when the spurned fiancé went looking for the ring with a flashlight.

Given Lois's hostile attitude and track record for hanging out with the wrong element, the Watsons refused to underwrite her plan to attend junior college for two years, then go to the University of Illinois. Wounded, she told her folks that if she couldn't go to college, she "wouldn't do anything."

After a year of sulking, Lois informed friends at a party one night that she had decided to enroll at the Evangelical Hospital's School of Nursing just north of Englewood. Even that decision was defiant: Her mother had once studied nursing at her parents' insistence and disliked the profession. She begged Lois not to go through with it.

But the next morning "some of the fellows" drove Lois up to Evangelical. Lois surprised friends and family—and probably herself—by staying with her nursing studies, paying much of her own way by babysitting. Despite repeated curfew violations, she graduated from Evangelical six months after Pearl Harbor and joined AAF's flight nurses program soon thereafter, drawing an assignment to Camp McCoy, Wisconsin.

Her mom and dad escorted her to the train station. "I remember Mom saying, 'You might accept sending your son to war, but not your daughter,'" Lois remembered. "My flip answer was, 'Oh, Mom, I could slip on a banana peel [here at home] and break my neck.'"

At Camp McCoy, she met a future bomber pilot from Kansas named Nolan McKenzie. Lieutenant McKenzie may have grown up on a farm, but he charmed her with the sophisticated ways he'd acquired as a member of the Pi Kappa Alpha fraternity at the Kansas State College of Agriculture and Applied Science (now Kansas State University). Like so many other couples during the war, they had a whirlwind romance, abetted by kisses stolen in Camp McCoy's recreation room, which Lois and her friends christened the "re-creation" room.

After a quick three months of dating, they bought rings on a whim and walked down the aisle of Camp McCoy's chapel on March 24, 1943. They had only a couple of weekends together as a married couple before Lois was shipped out to Louisville's Bowman Field to complete her flight evacuation training and get ready to serve in an overseas combat zone.

After they'd been in the air a while longer, Elna Schwant nudged Jens and motioned toward the windows on the right side of the plane.

"Mountains?" Schwant asked, incredulous.

Yes, indeed. They'd spotted jagged hills so imposing that the peaks were sticking up out of the clouds. The plane was over land, all right, but unless they'd gotten completely turned around, the ground was appearing on the wrong side. The heel of Italy should have shown up on the left, or western side. But the rugged mountain chain at which they were now staring had surfaced on the eastern side.

At about that time Abbott, sitting across from and a row or two behind McKenzie, saw another waterspout that seemed to hug the coastline. Thrasher and Baggs must have spotted it, too; they swung the plane back out to sea.

Where in God's name were they?

There was some speculation among the nurses that perhaps the transport had pulled a 180-degree turn and was back over Sicily. But that seemed too good to be true.

Now the cabin was getting truly frigid. Jens draped herself in her trench coat, closed her eyes, and tried to think of anything except being lost in a plane that was running out of fuel.

Apprehension was growing, McKenzie thought, but she was impressed that there was no panicky chatter. Abbott remembered attempting to keep what he called his "poker face," and thought most of the men were doing the same.

Major McKnight and their Bowman Field instructors would have been proud: The majority of the nurses and medics were maintaining textbook stoicism—at least on the outside.

But not everyone. Jensen glanced across the aisle and saw Paul Allen, the brown-haired teenager with the quick wit, shaking with cold and fright. It was Allen's second go-round with a violent storm thrashing his medical transport; a few weeks before, on a flight from Algiers to Catania, a squall over the Mediterranean had nearly torn up his plane. As Jens watched Allen wrap his arms around his knees in a failed effort to camouflage his nerves, she couldn't help but think of her seventeen-year-old brother back home in Michigan.

The plane again swung inland. Those mountains were getting closer and more menacing. The C-53 slowed down to circle something, reducing its altitude to two thousand feet.

An excited Thrasher popped out of the cockpit to announce that the crew had spotted an airfield. Everyone should buckle up and prepare for a tough landing; there was no telling what kind of condition the field might be in, he said.

One of the medics asked whether it was a "real" airfield. Thrasher replied that yes, they could see planes on the ground. Sure enough, Abbott and other corpsmen could make out what they deduced were Italian planes parked along a crude runway.

Maybe the airfield had been abandoned when Italy surrendered two months earlier, they hoped. Maybe, at last, they'd caught a break!

For the first time in hours the plane was filled with animated conversation. They started on a rapid descent that felt more like a roller-coaster drop than a smooth landing glide. Stomachs began to churn. Some of them gasped.

They were all craning their necks to try to glimpse the runway. It was hard to tell, but it seemed like they were flying into a dark valley dotted with dirty hills.

Just then they were startled by a stream of orange-red tracers, followed by a series of angry black puffs that exploded in front of the propellers and on either side of the wings.

None of the nurses and medics had been at the business end of antiaircraft fire. But they knew ack-ack and flak when they saw it. And they knew they'd been hit: A telltale clanking could be heard in the back. The C-53 now rocketed almost straight up as Thrasher jammed his throttles. The airfield, they later learned, was called Lushnjë.

Radioman Lebo burst out of the cockpit, whipping his head as he checked on damage. He muttered something about it being a close call and lamented the accuracy of antiaircraft guns, then disappeared.

A moment later, while it was still on its radical climb, the plane began swerving, desperately looking for thicker clouds. Clearly, somebody hostile was on their tail. Later the nurses and medics learned that two German fighters, ultrafast Messerschmitt 109s, had been scrambled from the airfield.

Under normal circumstances, a virtually unarmed C-53 would

have been easy prey for two Me 109s. But fortunately there was just enough fog to throw off the Luftwaffe pilots. Zooming ever farther inland, the C-53 was now surrounded by snowcapped mountains.

The nurses and medics had to begin contemplating the prospect of bailing out or crash-landing. Parachute skills had been taught as part of their survival exercises at Bowman Field. The school had proudly provided each MAES graduate with a personalized parachute; their names had been stenciled on their chutes just as they had been on their apparel. Alas, no one knew what had become of the Bowman chutes; they apparently never arrived in Sicily. It was immaterial; by now the passengers knew that there weren't nearly enough parachutes on board to go around.

A sergeant from Walden, New York, named Bob Owen began berating himself over leaving a contraband German Mauser pistol with a supply sergeant back in Catania. The moron will never know what to do with it, Owen complained to Abbott and anyone else who would listen. He'll trade it for something stupid. Or worse, Owen bitched, he'll lose it in a blankety-blank crap game.

It was classic sublimation. But for a minute or two, it kept their minds off their calamitous cirumstances.

CHAPTER 3

THE CRASH-LANDING— *AMERICANO! AMERICANO!*

They flew on for a half hour or more after their near-fatal stagger over the airfield. The clanging from the C-53's tail seemed to worsen. Shumway and Lebo kept slipping out of the cockpit to check for damage or ice on the wings, then slipping back in for more tense strategizing.

At one point the pilots abruptly turned the craft toward the sea and thicker fog, then, after a few minutes of picking their way through clouds, veered back inland. The next time Shumway came out, Abbott asked why the pilots had pulled the maneuver. Shumway said they'd spotted off the starboard wing four Messerschmitt fighters on patrol. Fortunately, the enemy pilots had not seen them—or at least so they'd hoped.

It was now past 1315. They'd been in the air for more than five hours. The situation was bleak. They had to be flying on fumes; the transport had been bucking headwinds. And now the ship was shot up.

They had all pretty much resigned themselves to their fate. The only way out now was to attempt a crash-landing.

But where?

The icy mountaintops must have looked like daggers stabbing through the clouds.

Abbott fretted that at any second the plane's engines would start to "cough and spit." They'd plunge into the side of some god-forsaken hill, never to be heard from again.

Orville Abbott was only about five-foot-seven, but with his thin nose and long forehead he seemed taller. His tousled brown hair tended to crowd his service cap. He could be outspoken and more than a little cocky. His given handle was Lawrence, but the guys in his outfit took one look at his middle name and branded him "Orville." After the war he went back to being "Larry."

Whether Orville or Larry, Abbott delivered his put-downs with such a crooked grin that nobody could stay mad at him for long. He was a young man of eclectic talents, able to fix things with his hands, retain them with his brain, and, for someone who had spent much of his adolescence in Michigan's great outdoors with a shotgun or fishing rod in his hands, remarkably well versed in politics, literature, and religion. Before leaving Catania, he'd slipped a prayer book into his musette bag.

Unlike some of the others on the plane, Abbott didn't easily rattle. Maybe growing up without a father had taught him to be self-reliant, to figure out for himself how to get out of tight spots. He also learned early in life to look out for members of his family, which suddenly consisted of twenty-nine others. At some point in their journey, Orville began, like Agnes Jensen, to discreetly scribble notes.

Not many twentieth-century Michiganders could trace their ancestry back to the pioneers who encountered wolverines in the wild—but Orville could. He was the descendant of an ambitious clan that built docks and bridges in Detroit early in the nineteenth century, then moved to the Muskegon Valley out west around 1860, when it was populated by more Ottawa and Chippewa Indians than whites.

Lawrence's great-grandfather Aaron Abbott threw himself into the nascent logging industry, running a sawmill near Slocum's Grove. Aaron's son, George, born in 1851, registered for the Union Army while still in his early teens but did not march off. George continued to run Abbott's Mill, which became more profitable as more settlers moved to Michigan. He died in his thirties from typhoid fever just as the logging business was drying up.

Lawrence's father, Aaron James, born ten years after Appomattox, worked at the mill as a youngster. Aaron James lost his left arm in a grisly accident; it was amputated above the elbow. A prosthetic hook allowed him to both work and imbibe alcohol, a habit in which Aaron James began regularly indulging.

The Abbotts sold their sawmill and moved the clan some sixty miles north to a Newaygo County lumber town known as Brohman. In 1913, Aaron James married Caroline, a woman seventeen years his junior. Despite her husband's struggles with alcohol, Mrs. Abbott gave birth to five sons in rapid succession: Lewis in 1914, Bernard in 1916, Walter in 1918, Lawrence Orville in 1920, and George in 1924. Caroline was so determined to have a girl that she gave her lastborn the middle name of Claire and proceeded to call him that for the rest of her life.

The rest of her husband's life, sadly, did not last long. Aaron James died from cirrhosis six months after George Claire was born. Caroline was widowed when Lawrence Orville was just four. She never remarried.

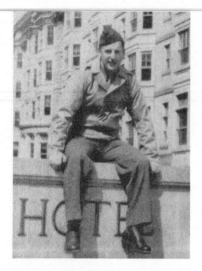

Orville Abbott during the war.

Orville ran a paper route, pitched in around the house, and, like his brothers, worked at part-time lumbering jobs to help his mother make ends meet. At age twelve, when Orville was out in the woods with George hunting small game, his shotgun accidentally discharged; he managed to shoot himself in the chin. He and George ran home bawling, but fortunately it was only a flesh wound. Orville's chin was permanently scarred, but the accident didn't stop him from continuing to scour the woods for deer and rabbit.

An avid reader, Orville graduated from Newaygo High in 1939. He moved to Grand Rapids and enrolled in pharmaceutical studies at what was then known as Grand Rapids University and is now called Davenport College.

In 1940, unsure of his career path in pharmacology, he joined the Army Air Corps, eventually volunteering to serve as a medic. Orville trained as an X-ray technician at an airfield near Tacoma, Washington. He enrolled in the officers' candidate schools at Camp Barkeley, Texas, and later at the Carlisle Barracks in Pennsylvania, before resigning to resume his medical studies as a noncommissioned officer. In the spring of 1943 he was sent to Bowman Field, where he was assigned to the 807th Medical Air Evacuation Squadron. The medics in the outfit called themselves "pill rollers."

All five of the Abbott boys served in the wartime military: Lewis in the Navy (beginning his stint in the late thirties) and his younger brothers in the Army. George, the baby, lied about his age and left school early. Bernard saw combat in Italy. Walter ended up in Army intelligence, stationed in, of all places, Cairo.

Agnes Jensen admitted later that, like Orville Abbott, she had given up the ghost.

"I just remember sitting there, thinking we would never get out," she said. "It was just a matter of time."

"Where are we? Where are we going to land?" Jensen asked her seatmate Schwant.

The South Dakotan flashed a fiendish grin and replied, "On the ground, I hope." Jens stared back at her, not amused by her friend's gallows humor.

Thrasher came out to announce that they'd found a field in a valley. "Buckle up tight," he advised, "because we're going wheels-up this time."

They knew from survival training that crash-landings on bumpy terrain were often made without wheels in hopes that the plane would slide safely to a stop. A crash-landing tended to deliver two violent jolts: the initial impact with the ground and a final thump before the plane completely halted.

Jens and the others reminded themselves not to unbuckle their seat belts until the last jolt had passed.

To avoid the mountaintops, Thrasher put the plane into an even steeper dive than the one over Lushnjë. Abbott's stomach was doing flip-flops; he worried that he was going to black out. He could feel his facial muscles "drawing into taut, hard lines."

Thrasher finally pulled back on the throttle; they began to circle at a low altitude. Below them was a big field of what appeared to be mudflats with a small lake at the far end. It was as good a place as any.

Shumway, the crew chief, had no place to sit and buckle up. So he stumbled aft and braced himself against the wall of the tiny lavatory.

The transport took another roller-coaster dip as Thrasher jerked the plane toward the ground. Abbott glanced out the window and saw the ground "sickeningly close." A second later he felt a "God-sent stall" that may have cut their speed by thirty miles per hour or more.

After all the talk of going wheels-up, at the last second Thrasher and Baggs decided the field was smooth enough to go in wheels-down. The decision may have saved their lives.

As soon as they hit ground, Jens could feel the wheels doing their job, bouncing along and keeping the belly of the fuselage away from a fiery collision. Abbott called it as "pretty a three-pointer [landing] as I've ever been in."

Wheels thrashing and wings creaking, the C-53 hurtled down the lakebed, luggage and equipment tumbling around the interior. Shumway, too, sailed through the cabin, his feet tucked under him like a broad jumper's. The crew chief, their musette bags, Hornsby's barracks bag, K rations, tin water pints, and a tool kit all went airborne and crumpled against the front of the cabin. After a few more seconds of screeching, the plane nose-dived into the muck, upending its tail, at least for a brief moment.

It took a couple of manic seconds before everyone grasped the fact that they'd survived. McKenzie felt sudden pain in her mouth and realized she was bleeding—and quite profusely.

"I looked down and there was blood all over my coat," she recalled. Later she figured out that Shumway's boot scraped her face as he flew by. Lois ended up with a split lower lip, an abrasion under her right eye, bashed upper teeth, and a permanent dimple in her cheek.

Everyone unbuckled their seat belts and piled toward the door. A stern female voice reminded them that first they had to tend to an injured man. Together, they helped Shumway out the door and onto the ground.

Only then were they aware that it was spitting rain—and that the C-53 was sinking lower and lower into the mud.

Fortunately, nothing was on fire, and there didn't seem to

be an immediate threat of the plane exploding. No one had to use the ladder; the transport had already dipped so low the bottom of the door was almost touching the ground.

They propped Shumway against the outside of the plane; the nurses fished out a first-aid kit. The women cleaned the cuts on the crew chief's neck and face, put some tape and gauze around a gash on his left knee, and gave him a shot of morphine. Lois and another nurse had ointment applied to their facial bruises.

Baggs and Thrasher walked through the muck to assess damage to the ship. One of the AAF mantras was that if you could walk away from a landing, it was a good one. By that definition, it had been a hell of a landing.

Slowly the group began looking around, trying to make sense of their surroundings. Everything looked brown and drenched. They had crashed on top of what seemed to be corn stubble. At first glance, they couldn't see any sign of civilization. The valley, such as it was, appeared completely blocked off by mountains.

Abbott and a couple of other medics joined the pilots, their boots sinking ankle-deep into the mud with each step. The C-53's wings had sustained a scary amount of damage from the antiaircraft fire. Copilot Baggs was affectionately patting the plane the way a grateful jockey thanks a Thoroughbred.

The land around them, Abbott wrote, "lay silent and brooding in every direction." They peered through the mist and concluded that an object on the side of a distant hill was probably a shack or a shed of some kind.

Thrasher, tugging on a cigarette, decided to round up a posse to investigate. They carried Shumway back into the plane, where he was joined by the nurses, nine of the medics, and radioman Lebo. Sergeants Abbott, Paul Allen, and Harold Hayes began trudging through the mire with the pilots.

After reaching the edge of the field, they had to vault over an odd man-made barrier of stubble and brush. They had just started up a steep wooded slope toward the shack when they heard frenzied yelling.

Turning around, they saw their colleagues waving arms and pointing. Their eyes followed the gesture to a hill opposite their position. A group of strangely clad men was working its way toward the C-53. The pilots' posse hustled back, beating the strangers to the plane.

Thrasher ordered one of the medics to retrieve the Thompson machine gun from the back of the transport. But then, thinking better of it, he wisely countermanded his own order. Offering resistance would only endanger lives—plus they didn't know who these natives were. Instead, the pilots chose the opposite tack, directing everyone to wave white handkerchiefs: the universal sign of surrender.

Now the locals were much closer, eyeing the interlopers as warily as the interlopers were eyeing them. The natives were cloaked in threadbare woolen coats and baggy trousers and seemed to be wielding axes and large knives—but no guns.

The Americans concluded they were farmers and shepherds. A heavily bearded blond-haired man appeared to be their leader. The Americans tried to use what little Italian or French they knew to communicate, but the natives stared back, uncomprehending. Thrasher asked whether they were German, even slashing the air with the sign of a swastika.

Some of the natives' heads began nodding, which caused muttering among the Americans, but it was unclear exactly what the nodding meant. Were they German sympathizers? Or did they merely recognize a Nazi symbol?

Another series of shouts reverberated across the field. A different-looking group of natives, carrying rifles and wearing oddly mismatched uniforms, was running toward the plane from the direction the posse had walked. They were bellowing something indecipherable.

As they got closer it was clear that they were grinning broadly and yelling, *"Americano! Americano!"* They had seen the white star on the C-53 and knew what it meant.

These new locals seemed to be dark, swarthy, and hirsute. Some wore fezzes and long-flowing capes; almost all were armed with rifles, some with ammunition bandoliers crisscrossed over their shoulders and chest.

A few were so excited it looked like they were dancing. One man grabbed Agnes Jensen's hand and pumped it continuously, repeating, *"Americano! Americano!"* as if it were an incantation. Many of the Americans, including some of the men, got bussed on both cheeks.

The nurses kept trotting out different phrases in different languages, hoping something would resonate. All it did was elicit shakes of the head. *"Italiano?"* triggered a violent head shake and a look of disgust.

The Americans, meanwhile, couldn't help but notice how heavily armed their new friends were. Some had what appeared to be hand grenades hanging from their belts. Others wore Italian military garb; still others sported various items from German uniforms. Many of their hats, McKenzie noticed, displayed a five-pronged red star, to which they would proudly point and say, "Roosh-a," baffling the Americans.

They knew they were off course, but Russia? That seemed logistically impossible.

"Jesus H. Christ! We can't be in Russia!" Thrasher swore.

Each American query was met with the same declaration—"Commandant!"—and the same hand gesture—a pointed finger in the direction of the wooded slope. A minute or two later, the commandant came galloping down the hill on a white horse, which the Americans surely viewed as a heartening omen.

Baggs strode out to greet the man. After a few seconds of discourse, the horseman clenched his fist, brought it up to his eyebrow, and acknowledged Baggs, who immediately responded with a crisp conventional salute of his own. The man dismounted and approached the group.

It was now pelting rain; everyone tried to huddle under a wing so they could listen to the commandant. The man could speak just enough English to make himself understood.

To the repeated queries of "Where are we?" he chuckled before volunteering, "Albania."

Albania? The nurses, medics, and airmen had all taken geography lessons as part of their training; most of them recognized that they'd somehow veered east across the Adriatic and were now a full sea removed from Bari or Catania. They also knew that Albania had been conquered by the Axis powers. Hearts sank as they realized they were stuck in enemy territory.

His name, he said, was Hasan Jina. He announced with not inconsiderable pride that he was the leader of a band of anti-Nazi Partisans—a number of whom were now gathered around the plane.

Hasan looked the part of an Eastern European guerrilla fighter: dark skinned, fiery brown eyes, an immense handlebar mustache, and a filthy uniform taken off a presumably now-dead Italian *soldato*. He spoke English with an accent that bordered on the impenetrable. But if he went slowly enough and didn't try to convey too much information in one gulp, he could be understood. His favorite verbal tic, Abbott recalled, was insinuating "never mind" into his statements, often at comically inappropriate junctures.

It became clear that Hasan believed he had unearthed a group of Allied airborne troops—the leading edge of what would be the long-anticipated Allied invasion to liberate the Balkans from Axis oppression. So *that* explained the big smiles and the animated kisses, the Americans surmised. Hasan kept inquiring about the cache of armaments they had brought with them, not understanding that the party was virtually unarmed. The Americans kept shaking their heads and pointing to themselves, repeating "nurses" and "medics." They weren't sure Hasan was getting the fact that they weren't combatants.

A moment later Hasan dramatically gestured, forming a circle with his hands, and distinctly said, "The Germans are all around!" He then explained how the enemy had ransacked their land and terrorized their people.

Thrasher handed the mustachioed leader a pack of cigarettes and declared that the Americans were in Hasan's hands. They would need his help to get back to Italy.

Hasan lit one of Thrasher's cigarettes, exhaled a long stream of blue smoke, and made it clear that they needed to move quickly. The Germans almost certainly had seen or heard the plane. Enemy camps were behind and in front of them, he gestured.

"You are *Americano*," Abbott remembered Hasan saying. "Good for us. Never mind. The Germans do not take you from us."

Italy was many days away, Hasan volunteered, without addressing the reality that they'd need a boat or a plane to get them there. Instead he would take the party to the city of Berat, a Partisan stronghold, where they'd be safe. There was a British general and his staff in Berat who could help them get to Italy.

British officers in Albania? That seemed too good to be true.

How far away is Berat? they asked.

For me, a two-day walk, Hasan replied. For you, about four days.

Abbott remembered medic Charlie Adams mumbling something under his breath about ending up in a rat hole of a country where it took four days to walk to the nearest town.

They returned to the plane to scoop up useful supplies, among them two life rafts, five parachutes, and the Mae West preservers. Hasan and his comrades, most of whom had never seen an airplane up close, were gobsmacked as they stared through its windows.

Three of the sergeants unscrewed a section of the bucket seats

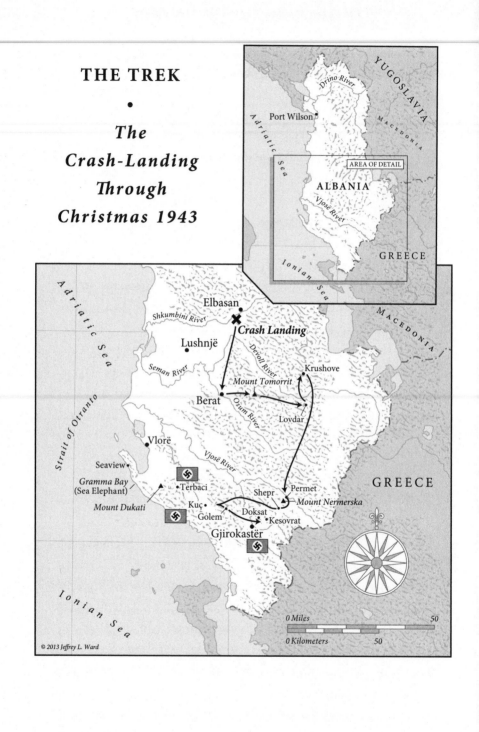

THE TREK

•

The
Crash-Landing
Through
Christmas 1943

YUGOSLAVIA

Drino River

Port Wilson

MACEDONIA

Adriatic Sea

AREA OF DETAIL

ALBANIA

Vjosë River

GREECE

Ionian Sea

Adriatic Sea

MACEDONIA

Elbasan

Shkumbini River

✖
Crash Landing

Lushnjë

Devoll River

Krushove

Seman River

Mount Tomorrit

Berat

Osum River

Lovdar

Strait of Otranto

Vlorë

Vjosë River

GREECE

Seaview

Gramma Bay
(Sea Elephant)

🗲 •Terbaci

Shepr   Permet

Mount Nermerska

Mount Dukati

🗲 Kuç•

Golem

Doksat

•Kesovrat

Gjirokastër 🗲

Ionian Sea

0 Miles   50

0 Kilometers   50

© 2013 Jeffrey L. Ward

to serve as a makeshift stretcher for Shumway, whose knee continued to throb. With Thrasher's and Baggs's okay, Hasan's men disabled the plane, taking their axes to the wheels. The pilots could barely stand to watch.

Shumway protested that he could walk. But he was told to zip it; they were hauling tail and didn't want him slowing them down.

Hasan explained that the first stop would be a "safe" village about a two-hour hike away. He insisted that Baggs mount the white horse, hoisting the copilot into an awkward-looking wooden saddle.

Off they went in the same direction from which Hasan had come, with Baggs and his steed at the head, Shumway being dragged in the middle, and Hasan's armed men taking up the rear. Hornsby lugged a barracks bag full of clothes and personal items; everyone else just had a musette bag slung over their shoulders, although Lebo was adamant that he should take the dead radio set. Hasan's men pitched in to carry the other supplies.

Their *thud-thud* echoed across the field as the little army headed God—or Allah—knows where.

The Americans were struck not only by how exotic the natives *looked*—but how peculiar they *sounded*. Albania's language, full of early Indo-European grunts and growls, seems harsh to Western ears. It remains today one of the oldest still-spoken tongues on earth. Descendants of the ancient Illyrian tribe, its people are proud to have been among the first inhabitants of the Balkans.

Hakmarrje, pronounced with a guttural "k" and a piratical "aarrj," is Albanian for "blood feud." The country's disheveled past has given its denizens no shortage of opportunity to invoke it. Ruinous warfare pitting ethnic tribe against ethnic tribe, religious sect against religious sect, southerner against northerner, has sadly dominated Albanian history. For centuries, paramilitary bands known as *çetas* (pronounced "chay-tus") stalked Albania's hills, their *komitadjis* (indigenous warriors) and *andartes* (guerrilla fighters operating near the Greek border) hell-bent on guarding turf, aching to live up to their *besa* (word of honor) by exacting revenge on one enemy or the other. Shielding Albania from outside invaders was usually less gratifying than settling internecine scores.

Albania has always been an abused stepchild, a rugged no-man's-land that separated East from West, European from Slav, and the Adriatic from the Aegean. What is now Albania was for a millennium ravaged by imperial hordes: the Greeks, the Romans, the Huns, the Visigoths, the Ostrogoths, various Byzantine clans, and—for five full centuries beginning in the 1400s—the Ottoman Turks.

When the seas turned disagreeable, ancient Greeks used the caves along the Adriatic for shelter, drawing self-glorifying murals on the cavern walls. Julius Caesar seized the area as a Roman province, but not before getting all he could handle in 48 B.C. from local tribesmen at Durrës and Pharsalus.

Conquerors from the Roman legions tended to leave the inland to the *çetas* and concentrated instead on exploiting the region's handful of natural harbors. Around present-day Durrës, the Romans built roads, aqueducts, libraries, and a massive amphitheater, which made the trade center a tempting target for seaborne invaders once the empire began to crack.

Still, lucrative trade routes were difficult to sustain; the natives had little to trade, and there wasn't enough traffic along the Adriatic. The Ottomans managed to sever Albania from Europe and convert it into what contemporary American journalist and Albanian descendant Peter Lucas calls a "Muslim enclave."

The Turks took a primitive country and kept it defiantly

primitive for half a millennium. A fifteenth-century rebel named George Kastrioti, who anointed himself Skanderbeg ("Lord Alexander" in Greek), tried to rally the Albanian people to throw off the yoke of Ottoman oppression. A lifetime of fighting the Turks went for naught, but Kastrioti earned a permanent spot in the hearts of his countrymen. It was Skanderbeg who adopted the eagle as Albania's symbol. All these centuries later, Albanians still call their country Shqipëria, "Land of the Eagle," and refer to themselves as Shqipetarë, "Sons of the Eagle." Albania's flag proudly displays a double-eagle motif to honor their mountain heritage. Nearly three-quarters of the country sits at three hundred meters or higher above sea level. Wild forests of oak, black pine, and beech dominate the valleys.

Sir Edward Gibbon, the English historian who chronicled the rise and fall of Rome amid Great Britain's own empire building, sailed past Albania in the late eighteenth century. Eyeing the hills tucked behind the coast, Gibbon observed that the civilized world knew as little about the southern Balkans as it did about the interior of North America. The region was seen as a remote Ottoman backwater, a crude place bereft of roads or cities or modern amenities.

Gibbon spoke for all of Europe when he pronounced the area untamable—a perception that remained unchanged even after Austria-Hungary began peeling off chunks of the region in the 1870s and 1880s. Well into the twentieth century, most Albanian peasants, especially in the south, remained obdurately Muslim, as Austrian-Hungarians, Greeks, Macedonians, Bulgarians, Serbs, and others—many of them Christian—rushed into the void created by the departing Turks. Albanians were so inured to outside invaders that it wasn't until 1912 that they officially broke away from what remained of the Ottoman Empire. The country's borders were finally defined a year later—but they didn't last long.

Upon the outbreak of the Great War in 1914, Albania declared itself neutral, but that didn't stop it from being plundered yet again. The war brought more chaos, as the area was whipsawed by marauding armies. Albania became, in the words of historian Miranda Vickers, "everybody's battleground." A hundred thousand Serbian soldiers died on a ghastly wintertime trek through Albania's mountains. Balkan battle lines were shredded as World War I unsheathed old grudges. In the north, various Albanian factions fought Serbs and Montenegrins; in the south, they clashed with Greeks and Turks. In between, the northerners, known as Ghegs, a substantial percentage of whom were Roman Catholic, renewed their centuries-old feud with the overwhelmingly Muslim Tosks from the south.

At the Versailles peace conference following the war, U.S. president Woodrow Wilson earned the affection of the Albanian people by becoming the first Western leader to embrace some measure of Albanian sovereignty. Like most of Wilson's postwar posturing, his effort to protect the integrity of Albania's borders proved illusory, exacerbating the conflict it was meant to avert.

Wilson's creation, the League of Nations, encouraged Albania in 1924 to adopt a parliamentary democracy, a bold experiment that—to the surprise of few Albanians—abruptly collapsed. The country's brief flirtation with the consent of the governed was led by Fan Noli, a Harvard-educated leftist whose government lasted a matter of weeks before being overthrown. Noli beat a quick retreat to Italy before taking up permanent residence in Boston, where he became a champion of Vatra ("the Hearth"), the Free Albania movement, and, eventually, an important Balkan intelligence resource for the Roosevelt administration.

Albania reverted to its autocratic ways, with quasi-feudal lords, tribal chiefs, and oligarchs butting heads. It was a testament to Albania's remoteness that it was the only Balkan country through most of the 1920s in which the Soviet Union did not bother to foment a Communist insurgency.

In 1928, a Mati Muslim aristocrat named Ahmed Zogu, who had led the uprising against Noli and then assumed a strongman role in the capital of Tirana, declared himself Zog I, king of the Albanians. King Zog, a Tosk, bought off the largely Gheg and Christian military establishment by giving each officer, regardless of geographic or religious roots, a promotion in rank, a hike in pay, and a spanking-new uniform bedecked with medals.

Zog proved a ruthless despot, ordering the extermination of rivals. He imposed such restrictive rules on Albania's "parliament" that only moneyed candidates loyal to his crown could afford to serve. The hardscrabble lives of most Albanian peasants did not improve under Zog's rule. When not squirreling away a fortune in jewels and gold, King Zog and Queen Geraldine cast nervous eyes across the Adriatic, where Italy's Fascist dictator, Benito Mussolini, was amassing military might. Throughout the twenties and thirties Mussolini forced Zog to sign one-sided treaties and banknotes, all the while making belligerent noises about adding the Balkans to an empire that now included Ethiopia and a large swath of North Africa.

Il Nostro Destino e sui Mare! ("Our Destiny Is on the Seas!") went a Blackshirt (Italian Fascist) war cry. Since little more than a hundred miles of the Adriatic separated Zog's near-defenseless homeland from Mussolini's, the self-anointed monarch knew he was in trouble. On Good Friday, 1939, as workers finished painting the king's summer palace on a bluff atop the sea near Durrës, Italian warships suddenly appeared. Mussolini, as an SOE report later put it, had "sent his army to foreclose the mortgage on his calculated loans to King Zog." Zog didn't hesitate: The king, the queen, and their trinkets escaped to Paris and, after Hitler's blitzkrieg a year later, to London. Zog never returned to Albania.

Mussolini quickly eliminated all opposition, suppressing newspapers and foisting a broadsheet called *Fashizmi* ("Fascist") on the populace. Even when the Italians renamed the paper *Tomori* after one of Albania's mythic mountains, the people didn't buy it.

Certain Albanian strongmen made their peace with Mussolini, even after Hitler's invasion of Poland. At least Il Duce was trying to build decent roads and rail lines from Tirana to the coast that the moneyed class could exploit. In truth, many oligarchs were more apprehensive about the unrest next door in Yugoslavia's mountains than they were about Italian repression.

A band of Yugoslav *komitadjis* had vowed allegiance to Communist Josip Broz, the charismatic guerrilla leader known as "Tito" who was trying to spread revolutionary turmoil throughout the Balkans. Early in the war, SOE hoped that Balkan resistance fighters, regardless of ideology, could put aside their differences and band together to fight Hitler and Mussolini.

Albania's Communist leader Enver Hoxha became, in effect, a junior partner of Tito's, managing with an iron fist an ever-growing network of anti-Fascist Partisan men and women.

Hoxha came from a prominent Tosk Muslim family that could afford to enroll him in the French school in Korçë, an academy destined to produce several other Partisan leaders. There young Hoxha won a state scholarship to study at Montpelier in France. He became radicalized by Communist agitators there and in the French capital. When he returned to Albania in the late thirties to teach at his old school, he immediately began organizing a Communist cell. In 1940, he gave up teaching to run a tobacco shop in Tirana, which in short order became a Marxist recruiting hub. Although no longer an educator, Hoxha still insisted on being called "Professor."

Despite his best efforts, Professor Hoxha could count in early 1941 only around 150 active followers. But Hitler's attack on Russia that spring made it easier for Hoxha to find enlistees. Soon hundreds of *komitadjis* were swearing oaths of allegiance to the Hoxha-led national liberation movement, a common front that included Socialists, Communists, and a few Anarchists.

Although Hoxha lacked Tito's charisma, he earned the respect

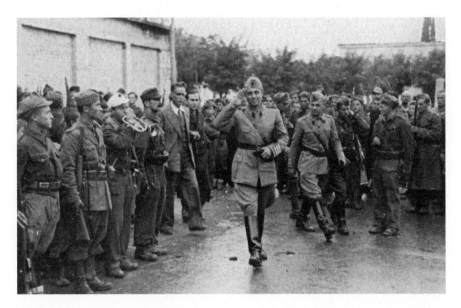

Partisan leader Enver Hoxha's triumphant march into liberated Berat, fall 1944.

of many SOE operatives for his capacity to mobilize and motivate. OSS and Washington, however, were less sanguine about Hoxha, Jon Naar remembers. Naar believes that the Americans never relinquished a deep mistrust of "Socialism," whether inculcated by Stalin's Soviets or anyone else.

Vdekje Fashizmit! ("Death to Fascism!") Hoxha's Partisans would declare upon greeting one another, which would trigger the reply *Liri Popullit!* ("Freedom to the People!"), accompanied by a clenched-fist salute and a pump to the heart. The first part of the exchange conveyed a sentiment to which most members of the Albanian resistance movement, regardless of faith or ideology, could subscribe. It was "Freedom to the People" that was distasteful to certain elements, known as "nationalists," most of whom came from Albania's privileged classes; for them, it made cooperation with Hoxha and his proletarian followers unpalatable.

The principal leaders of Albania's non-Communist resistance

groups were Colonel Muharrem Bajraktari, a former military aide to King Zog who organized a *çeta* in his native Lumë along the Macedonian border; and Myslim Peza, a regular army officer who created his own guerrilla band under Italian and German noses in Tirana.

Sundry nationalist and right-wing factions in Yugoslavia, Albania, and Greece refused to take up arms with the Communists— or in many cases, take up arms at all. SOE, eventually followed by its American counterpart, grew frustrated by the specter of the nationalists sitting on the sidelines or—worse—actively abetting the Axis occupiers.

By the end of 1943, SOE was concentrating the bulk of its Balkan resources on Tito, Hoxha, and other left-wing firebrands— all of whom were committed to fighting the *Fashizmit*. Four days before the Americans crash-landed in Albania, Prime Minister Churchill told the House of Commons, "Thousands of Albanian guerrillas are now fighting in their mountains for the freedom and independence of their country."

Churchill wasn't exaggerating: By November 1943, the people's insurrection was real. In the finest tradition of *hakmarrje*, however, Hoxha's *komitadjis* weren't just harassing Germans: They were fighting fellow countrymen.

It took weeks for them to fully appreciate it, but the Americans had crashed into Albanian anarchy. On a map, the country was barely larger than Vermont; its population in the early forties, moreover, was less than a million. Yet the situation was so convoluted that the Americans needed a scorecard to keep track of the combatants. No one gave them one. The whole time they were in Albania, the castaways could never be sure exactly whom they could trust.

They had no way of knowing it, but Hasan would soon be in touch with his superior, Rahman Runi, the regional Partisan head, who in turn sought direction from his military commander, Mehmet Shehu, and from Enver Hoxha, his conniving boss. The boss's order was to keep the Americans on the march from village to village. Hoxha wanted to leverage their propaganda value by convincing local inhabitants that the Communist network had an "in" with the Brits and the Yanks—and was facilitating an Allied liberation. By helping the Americans escape, Hoxha and his followers were buttressing their own grip on power.

The mud-spattered entourage hiked up the wooded slope for a half an hour before they came to the shack, an ancient stone building that adjoined a tiny cattle and oxen farm. Shumway was carried into a darkened room that reeked of sheep and goat manure. Their eyes stung from the fire pit that, sans chimney, was belching smoke into the middle of the room. Lieutenant McKenzie remembered stalks of corn and tobacco hanging from indoor rafters.

Outside Hasan was negotiating with the farmer to borrow a driver, two oxen, and an oxcart with two crude wooden wheels to transport Shumway and some of the Americans' gear. The party hung as many bags as they could from the spikes sticking up from the sides of the cart, then fell into line behind Hasan as they resumed their trek. Now and again they would encounter what seemed to be a faint cart track; the path would get a little less rocky. But soon the trail would disappear and they'd again be marching along choppy terrain.

Mud began seeping into the nurses' galoshes; their shoes were getting drenched. It had gotten so cold that some of the nurses took off their woolen liners and gave them to the medics, whose lightweight jackets weren't made for frigid climes. The airmen were wearing heavier flight jackets.

The group was methodically climbing a mountain, traversing one switchback after another. By now the wind was brutal; their clothes were saturated. They were famished; except for a cracker or two, none of them had eaten since dawn. Jens felt soreness in muscles that until that afternoon she didn't know she had.

It was practically dark by the time they came out of the woods and into a clearing. At its far end stood a squat, ramshackle cottage. A set of outside wooden steps led up to the second floor. The women were waiting for the men carrying Shumway to arrive before they set foot in the house.

"Take off your boots," the nurses said quietly as the men negotiated the stairs. "Why?" the men inquired. "Because we don't want to be rude," came the reply through pursed lips. Shumway, pointing to his damaged knee, kept his boots on; the rest removed theirs and walked in.

The room was tiny, about fourteen feet by fourteen feet, guessed Jens. But compared to the shack down the hill, it looked like the Ritz. A woolen rug sat on the floor. A rectangular stone hearth, again with no chimney outlet, was spewing heat in the middle of the room. Two small windows were open but did little to alleviate the smoke.

It was already feeling claustrophobic; it would get much worse. They huddled near the fire to warm themselves and dry their clothes. But the smoke was too intense. They'd retreat to the outer edge of the room for a few minutes—then duck back in.

Baggs and Hasan were in one corner, engaged in a serious debate over what to do about the plane. Hasan wanted it incinerated right away, before the Germans could find it, with the copilot arguing to hold off for a day or two. The contrast between Hasan's thick accent and Baggs's Georgia drawl gave their parley a humorous feel.

The chuckling stopped when Baggs asked Thrasher whether the plane should be torched. Thrasher was warming himself by the fire. He told Baggs that they had no choice: They had to destroy it. Otherwise the Germans would eventually find it and torture the locals until they got the information they were looking for about the Americans' whereabouts. If the wreckage were charred, the Germans might believe the passengers had died in the crash. Besides, the chances of the C-53 ever flying again were close to zero.

Baggs reluctantly agreed but told Hasan that the Americans, not Hasan or his men, would destroy the plane. The C-53 was truly Baggs's "horse," Abbott thought. Baggs—and only Baggs—was going to put it out of its misery.

They scrounged up flashlights. Baggs grabbed a flare gun and, escorted by Hasan's armed guards and four medic volunteers, including young Allen, marched back down the mountain. They lit matches and fired flares into the C-53—but the stubborn ship, soaked to its bones, burned some but did not go up in an inferno.

The torch squad returned to the stone house, where they found everyone where they'd left them: huddled around the fire and trying to make sense of what had happened over the Ionian. Dick Lebo, the radioman, explained from his perspective the sequence of events that caused them to lose their bearings. The radio went out; the Bari base radio operator had been unresponsive; the compass didn't seem to be working. As near as he could tell, they had crash-landed somewhere near the Yugoslav border. Big pieces of the story were omitted, like the fact that no one on the crew knew that day's password.

Everyone in the room understood that there was no percentage in playing the blame game. The flying conditions that morning were execrable; they should never have been given the go-ahead to take off; even a more experienced crew could have gotten off course. Still, the nurses and medics couldn't help but resent an aircrew that had grossly miscalculated and now had them stuck in enemy territory. They hoped the pilots would redeem themselves by helping them out of their mess—a hope that didn't quite pan out.

It turned out they weren't all that close to the Yugoslav border. They had crash-landed just below the Shkumbini River in south-central Albania, near the mountain hamlet of Çestie, a few miles southeast of a small town called Elbasan. As the crow flies, they were only thirty miles or so from Berat, which Hasan kept saying was a Partisan redoubt. But there were so many mountains between their present position and Berat that it would take multiple days of hiking to get there.

They didn't know it, but they had marched to a settlement called Kamuna and were now in the home of Tare Çerriku, an intimate of Hasan and Runi's and a fellow Communist commander. Five decades later, Çerriku's son Faik, who was about ten at the time of the crash, remembered the excitement in his home that evening. He distinctly recalled that one serviceman—Sergeant Shumway—was carried in on a stretcher.

Many in the American party never quite grasped the byzantine intrigue that convulsed Albania. On that first night it was a complete enigma. All they knew at that point was that they were hungry and tired. And that conditions were so miserable they couldn't completely burn their own plane.

Paul Allen, trying to be funny, asked when dinner was going to be served. He was told to shut up.

They heard a low rumble and went outside to check it out. Hasan announced that the British were bombing a distant German airbase.

Back inside, they were delighted when the mistress of the

house, presumably Mrs. Çerriku, suddenly appeared carrying freshly baked corn bread. It was the group's introduction to an Albanian staple—crusty cakes of grainy corn bread—that many of them came to abhor over the next two months. It was made with hand-crushed corn, water, and salt, all tossed in a pot and baked on the floor of the fireplace, protected by a heavy lid as it was smothered in hot coals. The corn bread didn't look very appetizing, but the Americans were so hungry that they devoured every morsel.

A few minutes later the woman returned with scraps of boiled chicken, which, given the locals' impoverishment, must have involved considerable sacrifice. The Americans profusely thanked their hostess and Hasan.

By now it must have been near midnight; they were exhausted. There was no place but the floor to lie down. The "bathroom" consisted of an aperture carved into the back porch: A waist-high partition barely concealed the hole in the floor. Urine and defecation fell where sheep and goats roamed, untethered. In Albania, barnyard animals often wandered into houses, which shocked the Americans.

Jens and some of the other nurses detached the hoods from their raincoats and used them as makeshift pillows. Lois McKenzie was already drifting off when Jens squeezed in between her and Lebo, the radioman.

As she tried to make herself sleep, Jens thought about an article she had read in *Reader's Digest* the month before about an American pilot who'd bailed out over occupied Europe; with the help of the resistance, he had managed to escape. She also thought about how distraught her parents would be to learn that she was missing. Jens took solace in the notion that maybe she'd get lucky and make it back to Sicily or Italy before the official missing-in-action wires were issued. They all dreaded the prospect of their folks receiving the awful telegrams. As the night wore on,

Jens got up to stoke the fire and make sure Shumway was doing okay.

Abbott, eyes smarting, moved away from the fire. He'd nod off for a few minutes, then be awakened by one of the nurses checking on the crew chief, who himself was drifting in and out.

Hornsby, the medic who'd thumbed the ride, was babbling in his sleep. When the corporal happened to yell out at 0600, the rest of the group took it as a sign to get up and get going.

Hasan walked outside and showed them how to wash themselves from a bucket filled with ice-cold well water. There were no towels, of course, so they'd dart back to the fire once they doused their face and hair.

Jens wandered outside and was startled to see several husky young women guarding the house. Rifles were slung over their shoulders; grenades hung from the waist of their coarsely woven skirts. Hasan explained that they'd stood guard all night. They wanted to meet the Americans.

The female Partisans came inside; through Hasan and hand gestures, they tried to communicate, but the two sides had trouble making themselves understood. The native women stared at the belted trench coats the American nurses were wearing and admired their visitors' hair.

At Hasan's urging, the women serenaded their new friends with patriotic songs. It was the Americans' first exposure to the intensely political agenda of the Partisans. Each song delivered chest-thumping propaganda, punctuated by a rousing cheer and a clenched fist tossed high in the air. Having not understood a word and still not quite comprehending the ideological impetus behind it all, the Americans politely applauded each number.

As the female fighters took their leave, the Americans began to worry that *way* too many locals were aware of their presence. Enemy agents would have to be oblivious not to know something was up.

Given the region's fratricidal past, it was fitting that the Balkans got a head start on the greatest conflagration in world history. Hitler's partner in crime, Italy's Benito Mussolini, conquered Albania five months before Germany savaged Poland. King Zog's desertion wasn't atypical: Few Albanians offered resistance to Mussolini's Good Friday assault. Italian *soldatis* soon controlled Albania's harbors and what passed for its population centers.

Mussolini, coveting Caesar's old Albanian prefecture, had deluded himself that he was restoring the glory that once was Rome. Hitler quickly disabused his partner of any grand scheme to annex Yugoslavia. The northern and central Balkans were critical to the Third Reich. Half the Reich's oil, one hundred percent of its chrome, sixty percent of its bauxite, and more than a fifth of its copper came from the region. The last thing *der Führer* wanted was Mussolini's adventurism disrupting his Balkan pipeline.

Angry that Hitler had thwarted his imperial dreams, Mussolini decided to plunge south. In the fall of 1940, without consulting Berlin, Il Duce sent a hundred thousand men—a tenth of them dragooned Albanians—hurtling across the border into northern Greece. The Italians were so confident of a quick conquest that they stocked up on silk nylons and condoms, the better to pursue a different kind of conquest.

The Greeks had other ideas. Fighting a skillful rearguard action, the Greek army snookered Mussolini's men into the northernmost chain of the Pindus Mountains, where they slaughtered Italy's lead divisions. Within weeks, the Greeks had not only recaptured their lost territory but launched a counteroffensive back across the Albanian border. By the onset of winter, the Greeks had the Italians reeling, seizing a stranglehold in the lower quarter of Albania. Even an Italian counter-counteroffensive in March 1941 failed to uproot the Greeks.

Mussolini's debacle could not have come at a worse time for the Axis. In late 1940, Hitler was planning Operation Barbarossa, the invasion of the Soviet Union. The Reich could not afford its southern flank crumbling as it tangled with Russia.

"We will burn out for good the festering sore in the Balkans," *der Führer* declared to his generals.

Hitler had committed, in the words of historian Joseph Persico, a "serious blunder." From the moment he first entertained world conquest, Hitler had planned to attack Russia. His appreciation of history was twisted, but he knew that if he didn't move in early spring, he would face the same fate as Napoleon and Charles XII—getting caught in the vise of a Russian winter.

In March of 1941, Yugoslavia's leaders, staring at the barrel of a gun, signed a surrender treaty putting the Germans in charge. Hitler was enraged a few days later when the Reich's puppet government was overthrown by Yugoslav patriots. Delirious crowds in Belgrade sneered at Nazi guards and spit on the car of one of Hitler's toadies.

Hitler was forced to delay his attack on Russia by more than a month as he cemented plans to carry out the Balkan campaign of terror the Germans called Operation Punishment. On April 6, 1941, German bombers attacked Belgrade, killing seventeen thousand civilians. In the middle of the melee, terrified animals from Belgrade's zoo got loose, galloping through smoke and fire.

The Nazi offensive lived up to its name, evoking the quick-strike blitzkrieg that had flattened France and the Low Countries eleven months earlier. Panzers, Messerschmitt fighters, and Stuka dive-bombers obliterated cities and villages. Inside two weeks the Wehrmacht forced Yugoslavia to surrender. Greece, despite the infusion of seventy-five thousand British soldiers hastily dispatched by Churchill, soon followed. By the end of April the Brits had abandoned Greece; once again Tommies had been pushed into the sea as they had been at Dunkirk and in Norway.

Hitler quickly made good on his pledge to eviscerate Yugoslavia. He tore the country into a jumble of states, some of which came under Berlin's direct boot heel; others were led by Fascist collaborators handpicked by the Gestapo. Hungarian, Bulgarian, and Albanian quislings were all awarded pieces of what had been Serbia. Hitler then appeased Mussolini by giving him Montenegro, western Slovenia, stretches of the Adriatic coast, and the southern part of Albania that the Italians had lost to the Greeks.

But Hitler did not trust Il Duce with keeping local insurgents in check. Hitler sent parts of two divisions to Albania to destroy the Partisans. Many of the soldiers were Bulgarian and Hungarian conscripts, not Wehrmacht regulars. Still, they were wearing the German uniform that had overpowered almost all of continental Europe.

For the first few weeks, the presence of Italian and German troops on Albanian soil appeared to keep meaningful resistance forces from coalescing. The Albanians, as always, preferred to settle internal scores rather than unite to fight an external enemy. But much of that changed on June 22, 1941, when Hitler sent more than a hundred divisions and some thirty-five hundred tanks crashing into Soviet territory. Barbarossa was not just an audacious act of treachery; it was, by far, Hitler's most lethal attack of the war. The Reich would never again have the capacity to launch such malevolence.

Tito and other Balkan Communist leaders immediately received orders from Moscow to strike back. Under Tito's tutelage, the Yugoslav Communists began training Balkan resistance fighters, including some of Hoxha's forces, in the art of irregular warfare; before long, the Communists began contemplating rapprochement with the West. The more powerful Tito and the Communist resistance became, the tougher the crackdown from Berlin. By the summer of 1943, Hitler had established *Generalfeldmarschall* Maximilian von Weichs, the commander of Army Group F, as head of the Reich's Balkan operations. Von Weichs was merciless in attempting to snuff out the Partisans. The Partisans returned the favor.

The Americans hung around the stone cottage in Kamuna that day, watching a parade of locals come by to gawk. On top of the stream of peasants and Hasan followers, at one point in midafternoon a well-groomed Albanian man wearing a business suit paid his respects. It was quite likely Rahman Runi, Hasan's superior and a key player in the Hoxha-Shehu network. The visitor sat down with some of the nurses and produced an English-Italian dictionary. Still, they had trouble connecting, although the gentleman was able to draw a rough map and point out where they had crashlanded, where they were now, and how far south they had to go to get to Berat.

Later that afternoon they heard a dull drone and realized an enemy scout plane was flying a reconnaissance mission over the area. They watched as it swooped across the valley where the plane was sitting, half-torched. The pilot could not possibly have missed it.

Between the local rumor mill and the snooping plane, there was now an excellent prospect that the enemy knew they were underfoot. The group recognized that it was too dangerous to stay in that location.

Hasan, in concert with a pair of older-looking men who had arrived on horseback, mulled over a scheme to wait a couple of weeks for the American men to grow beards, then dress them as natives as they trudged across the country. But that plan was rejected: They didn't have two weeks to spare.

That night Hasan and his band slaughtered a water buffalo so that the Americans could get decent nourishment. It was another act of Albanian generosity, if a grisly one. In full view of members of the party, the animal's throat was cut. Some of the Americans had to turn away, but others watched with steely curiosity as the animal was carved up for cooking.

It took a long while for the buffalo meat to stew. When the meal was ready, the Americans were shocked by the locals' method of eating. The meat was tossed into one big kettle with broth; one wooden spoon was produced. Diners were expected to get into line, plunge the spoon into the pot, take a few bites, then hand the implement to the next person.

It was so unhygienic that some of the medical professionals didn't think they could go through with it. But they soon learned to dig in, handing the spoon to the next person with a wry smile and a shrug of the shoulders. Most of the meals they had in Albania followed the same bacteria-ridden script, which no doubt contributed to the illnesses they contracted.

That night, Baggs again led a delegation of American and Albanian men to the downed plane. This time the C-53 went up in a pyre. Abbott and the other men watched the ship burn, wondering how they'd ever gotten into this fiasco. When they returned to Kamuna, Abbott recalled, the aircrew burned any item that associated them with the wrecked C-53.

Hasan told everyone to get a good night's rest. They would need it. In the morning they would be shoving off for Berat, where they could get more help. Being on the move was more appealing than sitting on their prats. Yet to the Americans, Berat and its "British general" were beginning to sound as fanciful as Shangri-la.

CHAPTER 4

SURREAL HEROES IN BERAT

The next morning, November 10, most of the Americans were up at dawn, splashing water over their faces and marveling at the rising sun piercing through the mist. Early on in their ordeal, nurse Jean Rutkowski tried to take a discreet pee behind some bushes, only to discover that privacy was an alien concept in Albania; passersby bade her good morning while she was still hunched over.

Albania's weather had gotten better. Worried that their cover had been blown and that the Germans could be in hot pursuit, the group was eager to get started toward Berat.

But first Hasan had to find them some mules. As they waited outside for what seemed an interminable stretch, Baggs took aside Hasan. Jens and three other nurses feigned nonchalance as they wandered close enough to eavesdrop.

Baggs was worried about the safety of the nurses and wanted a guarantee from Hasan that his men wouldn't abuse them. Hasan assured the copilot that he had already warned his men not to touch the women.

But what happens if they do? Baggs challenged.

Then I'll shoot them, Hasan promised, stifling what appeared to be a smile.

"I good friend to America. If I say I do something, I do it," Jens quoted Hasan as telling Baggs.

The good friend to America had, through a series of stern commands, managed to requisition four mules to lighten the party's load. Shumway objected, but the nurses insisted that the still-wobbly crew chief be strapped atop one of the animals.

Hasan mounted his white horse and led the group down a slippery trail. They had to march single file because the path was so narrow. It was getting warmer by the minute. Many in the group were wearing sporty scarves made from parachute silk they had cut up the night before. Now that they were on the move, spirits were improving, Abbott remembered.

With Hasan's armed guards keeping a wary eye out from the front and rear, they marched south for ninety minutes before taking a brief break. Soon after they resumed, they heard a dull whine. Hasan reined his horse and raced back through the column urging everyone to take cover: It was a German scout plane.

Crouching under the trees, the group asked Hasan whether he thought they'd been detected. Hasan assured them that he and his men always spotted enemy planes before the pilots spotted them. With that, the plane disappeared.

They hiked for another ninety minutes before coming upon a small settlement. The largest home had a stone wall that protected a vegetable garden. A swarthy man greeted each American with a nod as he escorted them into the house.

Three wooden tables had been set up in the large room with

the hearth. A group of local women had prepared corn bread and stewed chicken. The meat was served Albanian style, with a big bowl and a spoon on each table.

As the villagers giggled at the sight of these strange Americans, the nurses wondered whether the Albanian women had ever entertained a group of three dozen people before. Suddenly the enormity of the Albanians' sacrifice hit them.

How had Hasan signaled that they were coming? Where did these poor people find all this food? And how could they do all this under the nose of the Germans?

The 807th's flight had, by happenstance, crash-landed near a natural boundary that not only cleaved Albania north from south, but ideological right from left. Most of Enver Hoxha's Communist recruits came from south of the Shkumbini, where natives generally spoke the Tosk dialect and tended to be Muslim. The capitalist-supporting Balli Kombëtar and their counterparts in the Legaliteti, another Albanian national resistance group, tended to come from up north and spoke different dialects. A substantial minority of the anti-Communist guerrillas were Christian.

The Balli Kombëtar was bankrolled by Tirana potentates, big landowners, conservative tribal chiefs, and a few well-connected right-wing intellectuals. A hatred of Communism united them; they trembled at the prospect of Hoxha and his followers wielding power. Ballis didn't much care for Fascists, either. But some of them collaborated with Rome and Berlin in exchange for a degree of stability and the hope of preserving their riches.

On the other side, Hoxha had little trouble luring villagers with promises of getting them land and—at long last—sticking it to the Axis and their enablers.

With increasing support from SOE, Hoxha's Partisans were

beginning to enjoy success in harassing the Fascist occupiers, especially in Tirana and select parts of southern Albania. At Germany's prodding, the Italian rulers declared a state of siege, slapping martial law restrictions on the Albanian populace. Albanian police and Italian soldiers were now authorized to tear off women's veils to unmask disguised guerrillas. Peasants could not assemble in groups of more than five. Despite the crackdown, Partisans in midsummer of 1942 managed to destroy an Italian tank repair facility in Tirana.

Later that summer the first edition of Hoxha's forbidden newspaper, *Zeri-i-Popullit* (*Voice of the People*) appeared, triggering further unrest with its call for massive resistance. Soon, no Italian could venture into the countryside without armed guards. Mussolini's stooges demanded retribution, destroying hamlets believed to be concealing Partisans. Sixteen young Albanian women were murdered by Italian guards in August of 1942 for protesting the imprisonment of opposition figures. A few days later three of Hoxha's male charges were hanged for attempting to assassinate the Italians' handpicked Albanian premier.

In September of 1942, Hoxha and Yugoslavia's Tito, with SOE's encouragement, organized a conference outside Tirana, hoping the various Albanian resistance factions could set aside differences and fight the Axis together. The Lëvizja Nacional Çlirimtar (LNC), a national liberation front, was formed with the de facto approval of SOE under orders from Churchill. The issue of what kind of postwar government Albania ought to pursue was, at least by the Brits, held in abeyance until after the war.

The LNC's goal was to consolidate its support in every region of the country, especially up north, where monarchists wielded outsize influence. Its shrewdest military strategist was Mehmet Shehu, the product of a devoutly Muslim family and a graduate of the American vocational school in Tirana. After enrolling at an Italian military college, Shehu was kicked out for espousing left-wing political views. In the midthirties he jumped at the chance to fight Franco's Fascists in Spain, eventually commanding other international volunteers in a battalion of the famed "Garibaldi Brigade," Ernest Hemingway's favorite outfit in the Republican People's Army. SOE right-winger Peter Kemp, who fought with Franco, wrote that Shehu liked to brag that, in rapid succession, he had once slit the throat of seventeen Fascist prisoners.

It was pitiless anti-Fascists like Shehu who terrified members of the Balli Kombëtar, which got shortened to the BK, or Ballis, or Ballists. The American refugees, confused by it all, called them "Barleys." Some Barleys preached go-along-to-get-along collaboration with the Italians and Germans; more than a few were on the Fascist payroll. The longer the war went, the more reluctant the BK was to fight the occupiers.

"As resistance to the occupying forces accelerated, so the differences between the LNC and the Ballists became more pronounced," historian Vickers observed. The LNC, dominated by Hoxha's Communists, was pushing armed rebellion throughout the region; even those BK leaders not compromised by the occupiers wanted a less confrontational approach.

Hoxha's *komitadjis*, including Hasan's band, had to keep their eyes peeled more for Ballists than for Germans. By early 1943, the LNC had become almost exclusively a Communist/Socialist resistance network.

In August of 1943, less than three months before the 807th's errant flight, Albania's first organized resistance unit—the eight-hundred-person "First Shock Brigade," as Hoxha dubbed it—came into being. It was trained by SOE officers and men, armed with equipment and, in some cases, uniforms scavenged from Axis troops in North Africa.

Many women were among its ranks—a fact that never ceased to impress Allied intelligence officers and downed airmen. One Allied operative remembered their guerrillas' appearance: "[They] were of every age from fifteen to sixty. . . . They seemed fit, cheerful, and enthusiastic; sitting around their campfires under the stars they would sing of their courage and endurance, the skill of their officers and the wisdom of their leaders. There were some girls among them, who carried rifles and dressed like the men and whose functions, we were repeatedly assured, were strictly confined to cooking, nursing and fighting. Dress varied from town or peasant clothes to uniforms captured from the Italians and British battle-dresses."

The LNC's skill in making life uncomfortable for the Axis oppressors was rewarded in late 1942, when the Allies recognized Albania's independence. The BBC and the Voice of America began broadcasting proresistance messages—and providing resisters with radios to keep up with the latest instructions. Albanians who had never listened to a radio now began huddling around one at night, hanging on every word.

The campaign in Greece and Albania had dearly cost Italy: Nearly fourteen thousand of its soldiers were dead and more than fifty thousand wounded. Once Italy abandoned the war two months before the 807th's crash-landing, Germany had no choice but to move troops into the void. Hitler's First Mountain Division, the 297th Infantry Division, and a group of security battalions were summoned from Yugoslavia and Greece in late summer of 1943 under von Weich's command.

That fall, some twenty thousand abandoned Italian soldiers began wandering the Albanian countryside, desperate for food and work. Around two thousand of them ended up joining the Partisans. One of SOE's missions in central Albania was commanded by Major Anthony Quayle, a Shakespearean actor who later—in an exquisite moment of art imitating life—played a British special ops officer in *The Guns of Navarone*. Quayle remembered, "The Italians had been the oppressors for years, and the Partisans were not slow to take revenge. . . . Some were harnessed together like mules and for a daily handful of maize bread forced to drag the clumsy wooden plows."

Italy's surrender inflicted another plague on Albania: an occupying force that was even more genocidal. German assassination squads terrorized Albanian villages, exacting reprisals at any hint of insolence. Arriving with a roar of motorcycles, their henchmen would execute anyone—man, woman, or child—suspected of abetting LNC's bands like Hasan's. In the southern Albanian settlement of Borova, not far from Korçë, an SS hit squad shot in cold blood a hundred eighty peasants. Farther north, the Ustashi, a group of Croatian Fascists under the leadership of the notorious Ante Pavelic, colluded with Germans in massacring thousands of Serbian innocents.

The villagers who fed and housed the stranded Americans weren't just abetting the resistance; they were concealing sworn enemies of the Reich. The more the Americans learned about Albania's internal strife and its bloodthirsty oppressors, the more they came to appreciate the bravery of Hasan and his Partisan network of fighters and feeders.

The Americans thanked the dark-skinned gentleman and the tittering women for lunch, then went to retrieve their footwear. Two of their galoshes had gone missing—one belonging to Jean Rutkowski, the other to Ann Kopsco, a tall Louisianian. They looked everywhere—with Hasan berating both the native women and the guides—but the galoshes had clearly been pinched.

Sans the two rubber boots the group hit the trail, their muscles sore all over again. "The simple act of putting one foot in front of the other in the stone-filled mud was a chore," Jens recalled. The cheeriness of the morning hike gave way to stony silence.

After a couple of hours they came upon a stream that must have been the River Devoll. It was shallow—no more than knee-deep in most places—but bitterly cold and running hard. They had to be cautious. A slip could prove disastrous.

Shumway was still on one of the mules, which left three animals to help the Americans ford the stream. Hasan's guides rolled up their pant legs and hoisted the nurses—two at a time—onto the mules, then led the animals across by hand. It took three trips to escort the women. Most of the men waded barefoot, carrying their boots.

Abbott and Jens both noticed that Hasan's mood darkened once they reached the far side. The trail got steeper and more precarious. Hasan, looking perturbed, signaled for everyone to stub out smokes and zip their lips. His men kept hopscotching through the brush, relaying reports to Hasan as they worked their way up the hill.

Enemy patrols had been known to use the trail, Hasan soon explained; plus they were in territory in which Ballists were known to operate. The added tension contributed to everyone's weariness. By the time they came upon four houses carved into a hillside, they were spent. They barely had the energy to eat dinner that night, which was rice and corn bread.

Desperate for caffeine, the Americans realized that they had a few packets of Nescafé in their mess kits. They tried to make instant coffee by pouring water into their mess cups. But the cup handles were too short and the hearth fire too intense; they gave up after a couple of tries.

After three days on the trail with Hasan, the Americans now had a ton of questions about him, his organization, and his motivation.

He told them that he had learned English at an Albanian-American school run by the Red Cross and from an inspirational teacher named Harry T. Fultz. In the summer of 1939, following

Mussolini's conquest of Albania, Hasan left his village near Elbasan to join the fledgling Partisan movement. He hadn't been home since. No one in his family knew where he was or what he was doing—or so Hasan claimed.

They asked who was underwriting the activities of his guerrilla band. Eyes twinkling, Hasan allowed that he had a banker "friend" in Tirana. It sounded like this acquaintance would allow Hasan and his men to rob him from time to time as he transported German or Italian currency in his car.

The Americans were titillated to learn that their protector was, in fact, an Albanian Robin Hood, albeit one who appeared to be in cahoots with his "victims."

Albania was a corrupt place, Hasan stressed. Just about everyone had their hands out, playing the same slick game. The Americans could trust Hasan, but they couldn't trust every Albanian. They needed to understand that and be careful at all times, he warned.

The Americans sat, riveted, as Hasan described how he had become commandant of his little brigade: by killing more of the enemy than anyone else.

Hasan had developed a lethal modus operandi. He and his comrades knew the roads that German patrols were likely to take. They'd lie in wait in the woods, with one or two members of the party pretending to be in distress as they signaled for the Germans to stop. Once the enemy soldiers were exposed, Hasan and his men would open fire. They'd wait for darkness before helping themselves to rifles, grenades, uniforms, and ammunition— sometimes even the car if it were still drivable.

If the enemy soldiers survived the initial attack, the LNC guerrillas would take them into the woods to strip them of their clothes and weaponry. SOE officer Peter Kemp recalled that Albanian bands like Hasan's, wanting to save on ammunition, often slit the throats of enemy captives. The guerrillas tended to be such poor shots that in the end throat cutting was a more humane method of execution.

Hasan's *çeta* also perfected a diabolical method of attacking the personnel around German airfields. They'd hide in the bush waiting for an Allied air raid that they knew from underground radio communications was coming.

"Amid the din of antiaircraft fire, bursting bombs, and rattling machine guns," Abbott recalled of Hasan's description, they'd "pump lead at every Nazi they could catch in their sights."

To the Americans, these revelations were not only exhilarating; they were more than a bit sobering. They had come to view Hasan, as Abbott put it, as a "comic opera character," a voluble fellow whose broken English and compulsive "never minds" caused them to chortle.

Now they knew him to be both a thief and a merciless killer, someone who put his life on the line every moment of every day. Hasan was no longer a caricature. He was a guerrilla boss who commanded fear. Hasan "killed Germans like we kill pheasants back in Michigan," Abbott wrote after the war. "We began to find our friend Hasan not so funny."

The next morning, as they shoved off on day two of their march to Berat, it hit the Americans that it was the twenty-fifth anniversary of Armistice Day—the eleventh day of the eleventh month. The Great War had begun because of a tragic episode in the Balkans. And now they were immersed in another bizarre Balkan moment, spawning its own peculiar chain reaction.

As they got under way, nurse Helen Porter, from Hanksville, Utah, shared a story. Just before climbing aboard the troopship four months earlier in New York, she had visited a fortune-teller. The Gypsy lady looked into her crystal ball and predicted that, before the year was out, Lieutenant Porter would find herself in Berlin. The group decided that the charlatan had misread Porter's sign—that the crystal ball had actually said "Berat."

They hiked up a long slope until one p.m. or so, when they stopped at a farm dwelling for a quick meal of rice and corn bread. After they'd hit the trail for another hour, Hasan ordered a halt.

He gathered everyone in a tense huddle. A German airfield was nearby, he explained. To stay undetected, they would have to leave the path and conceal themselves in the trees along a ridge.

The woods were eerily quiet, Abbott remembered. Once they reached the edge of the forest, they were within eyesight of the base—and completely uncovered. Hasan had each member of the party lie still. Then, in ones and twos, he sent them scurrying across an open pasture about a quarter of a mile long.

As Jens skulked across the field, she glanced to her right. There in the valley about a mile away she could make out a small hangar, some planes parked in front of it, and a short runway.

Everyone made it across without incident. Their rallying point on the far side was a big tree. The Albanians were cackling with such glee that Abbott and some of the other men wondered whether they hadn't pulled a quick one just to watch the outsiders squirm. But the group didn't stick around long enough to see whether any Germans showed up. Hasan pointed to some garbage that he said had been left by an enemy patrol; sometimes, he told them, the Germans sent scouts to the top of the ridge.

The trail now became precipitous. After two and a half more hours they approached an enclave of four small houses called Pashtrani. There was plenty of daylight left, but Hasan announced that they'd spend the night there: Pashtrani was the safest place in the area.

They were now getting close to Berat, although it would still take three or four hours to hike there, Hasan said. That night's meal consisted of a little boiled chicken and corn bread doused in sour milk and again served collective style. The Americans were so exhausted they struggled to keep their eyes open, but Hasan hardly seemed fazed by the day's exertions.

Talk again turned to the dangers faced by Hasan and his men. When asked why the Partisans would take such risks to feed and protect strangers, Hasan explained that he felt the Albanian resistance had an obligation to help their friends—especially Americans—in the fight against Fascism. The people of the Balkans were still hoping that the Allies would come in large numbers to liberate them. Hasan wanted the evaders to go back to their countrymen singing the praises of Albania's Partisans.

Hasan, they would soon learn, had other reasons to ingratiate himself with the Americans—and was under strict orders to do so. The next day the group would begin to appreciate the propaganda value they represented to the LNC.

That night, they asked Hasan to tell more war stories about his dalliances with Germans and Barleys. Hasan admitted he'd had many close shaves and been shot at numerous times but had never been wounded or captured.

"If I captured, then I be dead," he admitted.

They woke up the next morning excited about the prospect of finally getting to Berat—and getting off the trail. The weather even cooperated: It was warmer and sunnier. There had been no rain for two days; the trail was less treacherous.

Hasan buoyed spirits when he announced that they'd be in Berat by noon. Most were upbeat and chatty as they moved down the trail in single file. Some of them, however, were beginning to feel the effects of an unfamiliar diet. They found themselves nauseated, sometimes feverish and struggling with diarrhea.

To rest a little, they began to take turns atop the mules. Helen Porter, the Utah native, was riding a mule that morning. The braids in her hair caused her Army Nurse Corps cap to perch awkwardly on top of her head.

After tramping for an hour, they found themselves on a ridge overlooking the same valley they had negotiated the day before. But now they were several miles south of where they'd glimpsed the enemy airfield on the eleventh.

As they maneuvered along the ridge, they were startled by a buzzing sound. It was distant at first, but quickly grew louder. There was no mistaking the noise: It was the sound of many airplane engines.

Suddenly there was great fear that they could be strafed by enemy fighters. They started scrambling for cover.

Hasan, grinning slyly, said no, he thought that the British were paying the German airfield another visit. A moment later the planes zoomed almost directly over their heads, flying low over the ridge.

"British, hell!" Willis Shumway hollered. "They're B-25 Mitchells!"

Everyone started screaming and waving their hands.

"They're our B-25s! They're ours!" a couple of nurses shrieked.

The bombers were so close it felt like they could reach out and touch the USAAF white star. They stomped, yelled, waved their musette bags, even tossed their flight hats.

All to no avail. The crews' eyes were zeroed in on the airfield, not the pedestrians below.

It was as if they had ringside seats to a boxing match. Jens counted twelve to fifteen B-25s and eight P-38 fighter escorts taking dead aim at the airfield. Two German fighter planes hustled to get down the runway and into the air as antiaircraft batteries swung into action.

Within seconds the flak was "furious," Abbott remembered, but it didn't seem to hinder the attack. The American bombs must have struck the base's fuel depot; a huge plume of black smoke darkened the valley.

As the planes departed, they again flew over the group's head, eliciting a last round of huzzahs. One of the bombers must have been hit; it was spewing smoke and seemed to drop behind the rest. The two German fighters never got high enough to challenge the crippled B-25. They'd only abandoned the runway to get out of the line of fire—an act of pusillanimity that produced much cackling among the Americans.

A USAAF chronology reveals that twelve B-25s in the 448th Bomb Squadron of the 12th Air Force, stationed in Tunisia, did indeed attack the Berat/Kuçovë airfield on the morning of November 12, 1943. OSS records, moreover, verify that Berat/Kuçovë was considered the most lethal of the six serviceable German airfields in Albania, with a well-maintained concrete runway and sizable fuel and ammunition depots. The after-action report noted that bomber crews observed two explosions and a fire near the runway. Flak was listed as "intense" but "inaccurate." After hitting the airdrome, the bombers then assaulted an Albanian oil refinery before flying back across the Mediterranean.

As the bombers vanished, the Americans looked at one another. Many had tears streaming down their cheeks. Part of it was heart-thumping pride and part of it was grief. Yes, they were almost in Berat. But now that their vicarious moment was over, they had to return to the unpleasant task of navigating a dangerous trail in enemy territory hundreds of miles from anything that could be considered safety.

The group plunged through a dense forest for another half hour. Beyond a rocky cliff, a valley came into view. In it was tucked a medieval-looking town; they didn't need Hasan to tell them it was Berat. The crystalline river and piney woods made Abbott homesick for the Muskegon valley.

Berat was much larger than the tiny villages they'd seen along the trail. An imposing castle that looked to be a thousand years old stood opposite them, guarding the city. Hundreds of homes were soon visible, as were a series of tall white steeples that the Americans took to be places of worship. The River Osum snaked between the hills.

Abbott thought Berat looked like something out of a picture book. The place was indeed old; its history was as tormented as any Balkan settlement. Its castle's foundation dated back some three centuries before Christ; the fortress had been ransacked by the Romans. It was then converted into a citadel by the Byzantine Empire and fought over for centuries by one invader after another. Berat had strong Christian roots, which explained all the white spires and its name, which derived from a Slavic term for "white city."

The Americans knew none of this as they trudged into the city along a bumpy cobblestone road. As they got closer to the walled city gates, they wondered why a big crowd had gathered.

Flabbergasted, they quickly realized that the throng was there to greet *them*. The Americans were being hailed, in the ancient tradition, as conquering heroes.

Albanians were weeping, trying to hug and kiss them, bleating, "*Americano! Americano!*" Their reception committee broke into song, including what the Americans later learned was the Albanian national anthem and a rendition of "The Star-spangled Banner" that was barely recognizable. Flower petals were thrown at their feet.

Creaky cameras clicked away, capturing the moment for posterity. The pictures were put to immediate use: The next day, photographs recording the Americans' triumphal procession were tacked up along Berat's only thoroughfare.

Many of the Americans' mouths were agape as they turned to

look at Hasan, who was beaming. The group's elation was mixed with dread.

How did these people know we were coming? And if everyone in Berat knew we were coming, who else knows?

There was clearly another agenda under way, but at that point, the Americans didn't fully appreciate what it was.

They were powerless to stop the euphoric wave, which carried them to the steps of a schoolhouse. Waiting there was Berat's mayor and other VIPs, who delivered a series of impassioned, if unintelligible, speeches saluting their arrival.

After a few minutes, a well-coiffed local gentleman whose English was much better than Hasan's began translating for them. It was clear from the orations that the people of Berat somehow believed that the Americans were there to liberate them.

Jens looked at her unarmed compatriots, limping from exhaustion, and tried to figure out how anyone could confuse them with an invasion force. Her eye happened to fall on Ann Maness, who, like Jens, had fastened two-inch bandages across her forehead to keep her uniform cap from blowing away.

This was the army that was going to uproot Hitler's finest from the Balkans?

Before they had a chance to question Hasan, he announced that they would all be the city's guests at a banquet in their honor. Despite their apprehensions, the Americans couldn't help but cheer.

The crowd swept them to the nicely appointed dining room of the Hotel Kolumbo, where male waiters delivered a sumptuous meal, served Western style (with plates and cutlery!). They supped on cold mutton, rice, potatoes, gravy, the obligatory corn bread, and the pièce de résistance, an entire apple for each. They were also introduced to an Albanian drink called *raki*, an almost colorless grape-based grog that, they soon learned, packed a wallop.

Eyeing the spread, medic Jim Cruise, a garrulous New Englander, opined, "These folks are going to be pretty damn disappointed when they find out we're nothing but a bunch of pill rollers!"

The party had just started for the pill rollers. After the meal, pie-eyed from the *raki*, they were paraded through town, triggering another outpouring of affection. Eventually they were led to a municipal hall council room, where more bloviating went on.

Finally, the hubbub died down; the people of Berat returned to their homes to recover from one of the most jubilant days in its history.

With Hasan out of the council room, the Americans were introduced to the gentleman who had been kind enough to serve as translator. His name was Kostig Steffa; they were told he would now be in charge of helping them escape.

Steffa was in his thirties, taller, chunkier, more cosmopolitan, and more Western-looking than Hasan. His mop of dark hair and mustache were nicely groomed; he was multilingual, able to effortlessly shift from Albanian to English to Italian to Greek. He also knew enough German to get by—a fact that, in the weeks to come, was to contribute to the unease that developed around him. He was, the Americans concluded after several days of observation, perhaps a bit too polished for his own good.

What would happen to Hasan? the Americans asked Steffa and the town elders. They were told that Hasan would return to his Partisan responsibilities farther north.

The Americans requested that Hasan be brought back so they could say good-bye and thank you. Hasan entered the room marching stiffly, as if about to receive a military honor, which in many ways he was. The Americans all thanked the Albanian for his courageous efforts.

Thrasher presented him with a parting gift: the Thompson submachine gun and its thirty rounds of ammunition that they'd been lugging around for four days. Hasan, they figured, could put the tommy gun to better use than they could.

Hasan had already displayed a flair for the dramatic; no one was surprised that he stood at attention while receiving the gun. His parting words were something like: "To you a safe journey. *Tungjatjeta*—I may see you again."

They had grown fond of Hasan and his dissonant "never minds." They were also quick to recognize that they owed him their lives.

The Americans were divided into groups of two and three to spend the night in different dwellings. None of them realized that allowing such separation was potentially dangerous.

Abbott and some of the other men ended up being taken to a bar a couple doors down from the hotel—the perfect denouement to a weird but wondrous day. There a colorful barkeep named Chris, decked out in a very American-looking flannel shirt and pullover sweater, plied them with alcohol. After Chris closed the joint, he invited them to his home, where the *raki* continued to flow. They whiled away the early morning hours solving all the war's problems.

The medics and airmen were trapped behind enemy lines in a strange country. Yet here they were, being feted as heroes and stuffed with food and drink.

As Abbott and his pals were hearing a bartender dissect Albania's troubled past, Jens and her roommate for that evening, Wilma Lytle from Butler, Kentucky, were listening to Steffa, their new leader, share *his* interpretation. Steffa lived in the most comfortable home they'd seen in Albania. It was two stories tall and had a potbellied stove that eliminated indoor smoke and provided steady warmth. A houseboy who spoke Italian dutifully waited on the family and their guests.

Steffa was cagey when asked his profession (it turned out he was the superintendent of Berat's schools), but was quick to volunteer that his wife taught elementary school. They had five children, the youngest of whom was three months old. His elderly parents also lived with them. Steffa learned English by attending the same Albanian-American school as Hasan, where both were mentored by American teacher Harry Fultz. But Steffa, from a more prosperous family, had been enrolled four years, Hasan only one. Steffa had also traveled throughout Europe, including time as a student in Rome.

Lytle and Jensen asked how the Albanian people could confuse their unarmed unit with an invasion force. Steffa answered that the Albanian people had waited a long time for Americans, their heroes, to send troops to liberate them from the hated *Germani*. But there are thirteen women in our party, the nurses pointed out. Albanian women often serve as guerrilla fighters, came the response.

Steffa explained that Albanians had always admired America, especially since President Wilson had spoken up for Albania at Versailles. Wilson and the Americans understood Albanians' hunger for freedom. The coastal village of Port Wilson had been named in the president's honor, Steffa revealed.

He told the nurses that if the U.S. and Britain would send more arms, the Albanian resistance would do a better job fighting the Fascists. Over supper, Steffa translated for his wife and mother, who peppered the Americans with questions about growing up in the U.S. and life as an Army nurse. They talked for a couple of hours, then delighted the grandmother by playing several hands of her favorite card game, fan-tan.

Steffa's wife led them to a small home next door that had belonged to Berat's onetime mayor, a man who had abruptly left town for "political" reasons, she said. What Mrs. Steffa failed to explain was that the mayor had been ostracized—and pegged for assassination—for his pro-Balli views. Had the Americans known how cozy Steffa and his family had been with an enemy collaborator, it might have caused more consternation.

But all those apprehensions were days away: For the first time since leaving Catania, the nurses had comfortable beds in which to sleep.

They snoozed until being awoken by Steffa's ten-year-old son, Alfredo, who meekly announced that breakfast was being served. Wilma and Jens drank chamomile tea and munched on goat cheese with toasted corn bread.

Things weren't quite as demure at Abbott's place across town. He and his party mates woke up with raging hangovers, which they had to nurse all day.

Nothing had dimmed the Americans' celebrity status. The group was taken by trucks and cars, mainly beat-up Italian vehicles, to a memorial honoring Albania's war dead. The shrine meant a great deal to the people of Berat, who turned out in large numbers at the cemetery. Steffa again served as interpreter as various speakers paid tribute to their fallen countrymen.

The Americans couldn't help but be apprehensive about being exposed in public. Any German sympathizer or spy—and surely Berat was full of them—would have a field day following such a large crowd.

With the throng in tow, the Americans went back to the hotel for another meal. There they exchanged a final good-bye with Hasan, who was leaving with his troops to hike back north.

After eating, the group one more time traipsed to city hall, where—much to their dismay—the speechifying started all over again. A man named Gino, clad in martial attire, down to an Italian machine gun and pistol hanging from his belt, delivered a three-hour stem-winder. The marathon oratory began, as near as Abbott could tell, with a description of Balkan cave dwellers. It then meandered, in numbing detail, through every invasion of

Albania over the next hundred millennia. Every so often Gino would stop to breathe, allowing Steffa time to translate.

But we don't want to stay here, the Americans were no doubt thinking while nodding politely and trying not to betray their impatience.

We want to get out of here. Please help us get out of here.

After the Chautauqua ended, Steffa acknowledged that the British officers Hasan had mentioned were not stationed in Berat after all. But Steffa did promise to get word to the British mission in Albania as soon as possible. The English could help figure out a rescue plan, he said. By now the Americans realized that Hasan had deliberately misled them about the proximity of the British agents to exploit them for propaganda purposes.

Had they been brought to Berat strictly for show? Could there actually be British operatives on the ground in Albania—and if so, where?

Those were the questions they were contemplating as they were herded back to the hotel for yet another dinner.

Early in the war, Britain's SOE was headquartered in several locations in London before finally settling on Baker Street, perhaps not coincidentally close to the mythical home of Sherlock Holmes. "Special" was infused into its title because it bore responsibility for an array of functions that Prime Minister Winston Churchill and the British high command regarded as outside the scope of regular military activities. SOE's first director was Sir Frank Nelson, an Asian trading magnate and a Tory backbencher in Parliament.

When European countries were overrun by the Nazis, those citizens who refused to accept defeat—soon dubbed "the resistance"—were forced underground. SOE's charge from Churchill and Nelson was to maintain contact with resistance leaders, encourage them to recruit and train saboteurs to cripple such targets as munitions plants, roads, bridges, railroad tracks, and telephone lines. The resistance was also tasked with forging escape routes for Allied agents and downed airmen, and with enlisting a fifth column of vigilantes who would, at the appointed hour, rise up against their oppressors.

As SOE evolved, each occupied country was given its own "section": the Norway section, the France section, and so forth. Even far-off Albania was apportioned its own section. The operatives in each section devised their own tactics but were expected to coordinate overall strategy with colleagues from the region.

Whenever possible, SOE required its agents on the ground to be fluent in that country's language and steeped in its culture, down to colloquial expressions and telltale mannerisms. But given the dearth of native Albanians in Britain and Egypt, where SOE did much of its MTO recruiting, that goal was nearly impossible to achieve.

With the number of Albanian immigrants in the U.S., the OSS had an easier time enlisting interpreters, analysts, and radio propagandists. Established in June 1942 under the mercurial watch of Great War Medal of Honor recipient William J. Donovan, the OSS's job was to coordinate U.S. espionage activities. OSS agents went through their own tough regimen, learning how to parachute at night, pick locks, forge official Reich documents, operate disguised radios, and assemble and fire all kinds of exotic weaponry. Prospective OSS agents were interrogated for three days by psychiatric teams, tested for their reaction to extreme stress.

It didn't take long for "Wild Bill's" agency to develop a thorny relationship with the SOE, although on certain big issues—like getting shot-down Allied airmen out of occupied Europe—they worked together quite effectively. Certain SOE members developed what Jon Naar described as an "inferiority complex" toward the Yanks and OSS: "They feared, with good reason, that the

Yanks would seize control over the strategic and tactical direction of the war on their way to replacing the British Empire as the world's preeminent power."

The Balkans remained throughout the war the province of SOE and the Brits, with the U.S. and OSS at best in a supportive role. By the spring of 1943, SOE had a sizable contingent of BLOs on the ground in Albania.

Operatives in Eastern Europe "carried out every conceivable type of sabotage so that the bombing effort of the [Allies] might be concentrated where it belonged—on Germany itself," wrote 15th U.S. Army Air Force historian Monro MacCloskey. Stationed in Brindisi and Bari, Italy, and working in close cooperation with SOE, OSS, the British Balkan Air Force, and, as the war wore on, the weather-impervious Russian Red Air Force, which also had a presence in Bari, the 15th AAF's 885th Heavy Bomb Squadron (Special) flew countless sorties over the Balkans, almost always in the dead of night.

Its name was a misnomer. Its pilots never dropped a bomb. Instead, it helped pioneer counterinsurgency operations, dropping liaison officers, arms, supplies, and instructions to Partisans in Yugoslavia, Albania, Greece, and a host of other occupied countries. In late December of 1943, Allied air forces, at the bidding of the U.S. commander in chief, would be assigned the highest of high-risk Balkan rescue missions.

Some members of the American party decided it was time to trade in their worthless—and suspicious upon sight—greenbacks for slightly more useful "Albanian Napoleons," as Abbott called them. Abbott and some others put their Albanian coin to good use in Berat, buying drinks and tipping waiters and bartenders as they were squired from place to place.

Saturday night, the thirteenth, they all went to a theater to see a propaganda film extolling Greece's 1941 victory over Italian troops in the mountains of southern Albania. Little did they know that in a matter of days they'd be marching through those same hills.

Jens and Lytle again were paired for that evening, but this time in a different home, although one comparably upscale to Steffa's. After a supper of mutton stew, the ladies were served a sweet Turkish coffee in demitasse cups. They complimented their hostess on her china. Many Berat families had hidden their family heirlooms, she explained. If the Germans ever decided to take Berat, they would loot every home for anything valuable. They would, moreover, seize hostages and threaten to kill them if they didn't obtain complete cooperation.

The Gestapo had taken away hostages from a nearby town two years before; the hostages still had not returned and were feared dead.

"That's why we have no faith in the word of Germans," their host said.

When his wife led them to a bedroom with a fluffy feather mattress, she apologized about not having an extra blanket. But with an air of resignation she said that if there were an extra blanket, the Germans would just steal it when they got to Berat.

The next morning, Sunday, November 14, the Americans got to sleep in a little. Several members of the group attended church with their host families, which pleased the villagers no end.

That afternoon, the group was taken to the old castle and given a rambling lesson on the city's Roman legacy. As they returned to town, they visited a hospital and a barracks that housed Partisan soldiers. They were also ushered to a cemetery in which fallen Italian pilots had been buried. The Americans were perplexed by gravestones that included propellers or other parts of the wrecked plane, as well as photos of the pilot's corpse. It was a peculiar way, the Americans thought, to pay homage to enemy airmen.

As they made their rounds through the streets, the people of Berat would greet them with the anti-Fascist salute and the *Vdekje Fashizmit! Liri Popullit!* exchange. It grew so tiresome that Abbott and his buddies started muttering in response, "And to hell with you!" punctuated with a dismissive wave of the right arm.

The Americans may have grown tired of the ritualistic greeting, but they certainly hadn't grown tired of the ritualistic toasting in their honor. On Sunday afternoon, the wine and *raki* again flowed freely. Some of them were tipsy when they were taken back to the theater for that evening's entertainment. Instead of a movie, they were treated to a musical performance by young people. The star of the show was a handsome lad who had given up his college studies to come to Berat to fight the Italians a couple of years earlier. Now he was fighting a different enemy.

Jens's roommate for the evening was Ann Kopsco. No one in the house spoke English, which was fine by the Americans, because they couldn't wait to get to bed. Unfortunately, their mattress practically sagged to the floor. Still, they had no trouble getting to sleep.

Abbott and John "J.P." Wolf from Milwaukee were quartered together that night. As they drifted off to sleep, they were chuckling over their surreal couple of days in Berat. There were a lot worse ways to spend the war than being hailed as conquering heroes.

"They could leave us right here for the duration without making me too sore," Wolf joked.

CHAPTER 5

SEPARATION—
THE GERMANS ATTACK

It was barely dawn when they heard the first muffled roar. Most of the Americans were still in bed, some suffering the effects of too much *raki* and revelry.

At first they didn't know what to make of it. It might have been thunder. Or maybe a distant air attack.

But then an unmistakable *boom! boom!* caused them to bolt upright. An instant later they were scrambling for their clothes. As they rushed to get dressed, Wolf and Abbott speculated that it could have been Barleys and the Partisans skirmishing. But as the medics' heads cleared, they remembered that neither the LNC nor the BK was likely to have artillery. And they definitely didn't have tanks.

Their Albanian host at that instant came running into the room shrieking in broken English about Germans attacking and Partisans defending and telling them to run, run!

Across town, Jensen and Kopsco fell out of their sagging mattress, threw on their blouses and slacks, and raced toward the front door. Their hosts, who spoke no English, were peering out the doorway, kneading their hands and murmuring prayers and imprecations. The people of Berat were living the nightmare they had dreaded for years.

Kopsco and Jensen were trying to figure out from what direction the cannon fire was coming when two of the sergeants burst into view. The medics told them they were heading toward the hotel to find out what the pilots wanted to do. They promised to double back to fill in Jens and Kopsco.

The two nurses ran back into the house to get their coats and grab their musette bags. Their hosts pointed to an already laid-out breakfast table, but the nurses shook their heads, apologized, thanked them once more, and kept moving.

Bedlam reigned. The *boom! boom!* had been supplanted by the *rat-a-tat-tat!* of small-arms fire.

It was so close it was terrifying. Berat was in full-throated panic.

"[The people] were moving out, using everything on wheels they could push or pull, vehicles piled high with bedclothes, clocks, chairs, pots and pans, crocks, bulging bags of all sizes," Abbott remembered. "There were old men and old women struggling with heavy loads, tears streaming down from their faces. Mothers moved along with babies in their arms and squalling children clinging to their skirts."

Rifles in hand, grim-faced militia members, many women among them, were double-timing toward the noise.

Above the din, the malevolent hum of warplanes could be heard. The Americans at that point couldn't see the aircraft, but they knew they were out there, lurking.

The sergeants came back to Jens and Kopsco, hollering that the pilots wanted the entire group at the hotel right away. Trucks to take them out of town were supposed to be meeting them there at any instant, they said.

The Americans threaded their way through the tumult. A human flood was now bursting in both directions along Berat's only real street.

Wolf and Abbott ran into Sergeant Charles Zeiber. The three of them muscled through the crowd. They saw a barefooted older woman, eyes glazed, carrying a glass pitcher in one hand and a batch of clothes in the other.

Suddenly the gunfire stopped, which the scrambling Americans did not view as a positive sign. Maybe the Partisan defense had collapsed and the Germans were surging into town.

Amid the pandemonium, Sergeant Bob Owen had managed to mount a horse. Coming toward the hotel and the nearby city hall from different directions, Jens, Kopsco, Zeiber, Abbott, and Wolf all spotted Owen perched above the writhing sea of humanity. Owen was trying to bark instructions—and so were the pilots.

Having spent the night at the hotel, Baggs, Thrasher, and several nurses were frantically signaling three or four small trucks that had just pulled up, scattering people in their path. The trucks had been stolen months before from the woebegone Italian army and looked it: They were barely running. But they must have seemed like limousines to the Americans.

Kostig Steffa, along with some rifle-wielding Albanians whom they didn't recognize, was clearing people out of the way and yelling at the Americans to get into the trucks. Owen stayed on his horse and, after a shouted word from Thrasher, reined it toward a road running up a hillside opposite the firing.

Zeiber, Abbott, and Wolf piled into a truck, desperately counting heads in their vehicles and the others. Harold Hayes caught their eye and declared it was "the Fourth of July in Technicolor."

Had all thirty Americans made it to the hotel? It didn't seem like it.

Jens and Kopsco were still up the street when the caravan, led by Owen's horse, jerked into traffic. Thrasher reached out of one truck and scooped the two nurses aboard. The vehicle was packed to the gills. The Americans were craning their necks, trying to account for everyone in the party. Jens's eyes fell on Steffa, sitting inert in the truck in front of hers. He looked "like a scared little rabbit," she recalled.

Given Steffa's assured demeanor of the past three days, she was surprised that he was so shaken. *Hadn't Berat's resistance prepared for this moment?*

Thrasher pointed to the road up the hill and hollered for the driver to follow Owen and his horse. Hundreds of petrified refugees joined the retreat. It was slow going. The road was narrow and choked with people. It would have been quicker to get out and jog, which several members of the party proceeded to do.

The caravan went less than half a mile up the hill before the lead driver slammed on the brakes. Passersby were screaming and pointing to the sky. Having understood the threat, Owen was trying to drag his braying horse into the woods.

They all poured out of the trucks, diving for cover in every direction while trying to eyeball the German planes. Abbott figured the farther away from the road and its knot of refugee targets he could get, the better. So he sprinted a hundred yards or more through the forest before realizing that Gilbert Hornsby and J. P. Wolf were only a few steps behind.

It took the trio a while to get their bearings; panting heavily, they knelt down. They counted three, maybe four Stuka dive-bombers screeching overhead. At that moment, the enemy pilots seemed more intent on bombing the town than strafing its refugees. But that could change at any instant.

Jens grabbed Baggs in a different spot in the woods and asked whether the other nurses and medics had been accounted for. Baggs told her he didn't know everyone's name, let alone their whereabouts, which was not the message Jens wanted to hear. The artillery fire that had died down again erupted.

The American evaders were spread all over the hill; so were hundreds of Albanians. Steffa and some others began hollering for the Americans to get back on the trucks—a curious order given the proximity of hostile aircraft. Some jumped back into the vehicles. Others hustled by foot toward the top of the hill.

It took an excruciating five minutes to reload the trucks, but eventually they lurched forward. People were hanging off the sides, anxiously looking over the trees for the planes. They went only a couple hundred yards before the ungodly noise erupted again. The trucks came to such an abrupt halt that people were tossed onto the ground.

This time Thrasher yelled for everyone to stay off the road and make themselves less of a target. He pointed to some brush beyond a grassy field a quarter mile or so farther up the hill and screamed at everyone within earshot to reconnoiter there.

But not everyone heard him. Somehow in the confusion the Americans got separated. Seventeen of them, including Jens and Thrasher, got to the brushy area, hiding in the weeds with scores of Albanians.

A few hundred yards farther up and around the slope, near a deserted Christian chapel, Steffa, Abbott, and nine other Americans watched a Partisan machine gunner fire at the enemy planes before finally realizing it was futile.

Abbott heard a different-sounding noise, looked up, and spotted two Me 109s bearing down on Berat, guns blazing. Now there were three or four dive-bombers and two fighter planes terrorizing a virtually defenseless town.

Jens, farther down the hill, looked around for Steffa but couldn't find him in the turmoil. A teenage boy wearing an Italian army uniform was following the planes with a pair of binoculars. The boy wordlessly shared the field glasses with Thrasher.

In a few seconds, no one's eyes needed extra help. The enemy pilots were stalking targets at the base of the hill. Given the hill's slope, most of the Americans couldn't quite see the trucks they'd abandoned. But the jarring sound of metal on metal suggested that the planes had scored a direct hit.

Willis Shumway, still nursing his bad leg (by then he was calling himself "Old Step-and-a-Half"), had been able to get only a few yards away from the trucks. Facedown in the dirt, he counted four separate strafing passes, the bullets whizzing all around. Miraculously, he wasn't hit.

A few minutes later, the Nazi planes disappeared over the mountains, leaving Berat wrecked and smoldering.

Shumway limped up the hill and was hailed by Abbott's group. No one was sure what to do or where to go. Separated by only a few hundred yards, the two groups never connected. The contingent with Steffa and Abbott began marching east, toward a pass between two mountaintops.

Jens's larger retinue stayed put, at least for a few minutes. The teenage boy near Thrasher and Baggs was looking through his field glasses, trying to assess the damage that had been inflicted on the village. Suddenly he began pointing and cursing as he handed the binoculars to Baggs. A tank was chugging down Berat's one street, trailed by half-tracks and infantry. The enemy armored unit was clearly heading toward the refugees' position. Within seconds, the tank started up the hillside.

Abbott's group, although farther away, saw and heard the tank, too. Steffa urged them to take cover. Continuing to move would only present the tank with an easier target. They hid in the trees and waited.

The *Panzerkampfwagen* sat at the bottom of the hill for a good ten minutes. No soldier climbed out of its hatch. The half-tracks and the infantrymen stayed between the tank and the town.

Abbott watched, dumbfounded, as Lieutenant Paula Kanable spent the time waiting on the tank to powder her face. Sitting cross-legged behind a tree, the former airline stewardess pulled out a mirror and makeup kit, dabbing on eyeliner and lipstick as a Nazi armored unit growled a quarter of a mile away.

By then the Americans had heard enough from Hasan to know that the last thing German soldiers stationed in Albania wanted was to wander too far into the mountains and be ambushed. The enemy troops turned and headed back to the burning village, where the families that had been housing and feeding the Americans for the past three days were now at the mercy of Fascist conquerors.

Steffa, having left behind his wife, his parents, and his five children, stood up as the tank moved off, clapped his hands, and urged the Americans to pull out and begin marching away from town.

But what of the others? the Americans protested. *And where was he taking them?*

He assured them that the others would be heading toward the same safe destination. The group was being led by one of his men. They would be fine, he promised.

The Americans weren't so sure. None of them liked the idea of being separated. They kept goosing their necks, hoping their comrades would come into sight.

After several more minutes of tense back-and-forth, they decided they had no choice. They were down to bare-bones supplies. With the Nazis now in control of Berat, they couldn't head that direction. And they certainly couldn't wander around the hills by themselves.

Steffa and his guides led them to a sinewy mountain trail. With Steffa and Abbott were lieutenants Kanable, Gertrude "Tooie"

Dawson, Ann "Markie" Markowitz, and Jean Rutkowski, plus sergeants Paul Allen, Willis Shumway, Robert Cranson, and J. P. Wolf, as well as Corporal Gilbert Hornsby.

On the way up the hill, Markie sarcastically revealed that it was her birthday. All agreed that she'd been given a hell of a birthday gift. In spite of everything that had happened, they wished her many happy returns.

Farther down and around the hill, still out of the other group's sight line, Jens's assemblage was going through a similar debate, now that the immediate threat of the tank had waned.

Where did they need to go? How could they reunite with the other group?

They found themselves listening to the Albanian boy in the Italian army uniform. He introduced himself as "Szhanny," which they took as a Balkan version of "Johnny." His English was not good, but he kept pointing over his shoulder, excitedly repeating the name of a village he wanted to take them to. The Americans asked about the whereabouts of the other group, but it wasn't clear he understood.

Looking around, they realized that thirteen members of the party were missing. The nurses began counting on their fingers.

Markowitz, Rutkowski, Kanable, and Dawson had all been on the trucks or the road with them an hour before and were hopefully with the other group. No one could recall seeing Wilma Lytle, Ann Maness, or Helen Porter that morning.

Seven of the thirteen women could not be accounted for; nor could six of the seventeen men. The gravity of the situation hit them; they were all worried sick. But they couldn't go down the hill to look for them. If they were caught, that would mean almost certain torture, since their pictures were plastered all over Berat.

The Germans would surely accuse them of espionage and might shoot them and anyone who helped them, just to let the Albanian populace know the consequences of collaboration.

The Americans had no choice but to follow "Johnny" into the hills and hope for the best. He couldn't have been more than fourteen or fifteen years old, they reckoned. They couldn't tell if he was Italian or Albanian or what. And they were putting their lives in his hands!

Following the teenager were lieutenants Jensen, Lois Watson McKenzie, Ann Kopsco, Elna Schwant, Lillian "Tassy" Tacina, and Frances Nelson, plus lieutenants Thrasher and Baggs and sergeants Dick Lebo, Charlie Zeiber, Charlie Adams, Jim Cruise, Raymond Eberg, Harold Hayes, Bill Eldridge, and Gordon MacKinnon.

By now it was past noon. Steffa led the Abbott group up a mountain trail. The only food they'd eaten all day was a batch of anchovies given them by a kindly Italian officer who hid with them during the strafing. At around three o'clock, they reached a settlement that had become a rallying point for wayward Italians. A machine gun nest manned by a half dozen *soldati* guarded the valley side of the village.

They were greeted by a distinguished-looking colonel, who exchanged pleasantries in Italian with Steffa before formally saluting each of the Americans. The colonel dispatched aides to fetch them some food. He had not seen the other American group, he told Steffa.

The soldiers produced several loaves of wheat bread and some eggs and anchovies. Abbott and Wolf pocketed their eggs, hoping to scramble them later. Somehow the colonel also produced a mule, on which they put Shumway and their meager supplies.

After a break of twenty minutes, they headed back up the

mountain, toward a village that would be safer than the one they had just visited, Steffa assured them. He was convinced that the other group was only a few minutes behind. The Americans were skeptical, but kept plowing forward.

As they got deeper into the hills, they got a chance to ask Steffa why the Germans had attacked Berat the way they did. Steffa's best guess was that Ballist leaders had told the Germans that the town had become a Partisan stronghold.

Had the Germans known that the stranded Americans were in Berat? Steffa didn't think so—but didn't assuage their fears, saying in the next breath that the Germans would certainly know now that they were in the nearby hills.

At this point, the Americans didn't know what to believe. But they knew this much: The Berat propaganda parade engineered by Hasan and Steffa was coming back to haunt the very people it was meant to celebrate.

Jens and her comrades slogged for some five hours without food. Finally they, too, approached a village, this one with just three dwellings. Only Albanians were present, no Italians, so it's not likely that this village was the same one in which the other group had stopped. Jens's contingent at that point was probably on a different trail on a different side of the mountain.

Johnny questioned a village elder, then announced that they would be spending the night there. It took Johnny a while, but through a series of gestures he indicated that they would split up and sleep in all three houses.

"No!" they all shouted.

They'd learned from their mistake the night before. They would all spend the night together in the event of another German or Ballist attack, even if that meant no beds and extreme discomfort.

All seventeen huddled in a room even more cramped and dingy than where they spent their first night in Kamuna. It seemed a lifetime, but it had been only a week.

The day's trauma and the lack of food cast a pall as, poking at a smoky fire, they tried to get some rest. They couldn't help but think that their friends and host families had met a ghastly fate, and that, at any moment, they could join them.

Jens remembered Lois, who reveled in playing devil's advocate, cheerily reminding the group that evening of their Bowman Field survival training: If captured, offer the enemy only name, rank, and serial number. Lois's great pal Fran Nelson chided McKenzie for being so gloomy. But the tête-à-tête made them realize that they needed to destroy any personal items that might give the Germans a hint as to where they had come from or their family lives back home.

Into the fire they tossed half-written letters, pictures, postcards, and anything else incriminating. Someone in Berat had taken a photograph of Jens and Ann Maness as they entered the city, grinning goofily with their hats held in place by Band-Aids. Jens thought it made them look a little like Jacob Marley haunting Scrooge on Christmas Eve. Her heart was heavy as she tossed the picture into the hearth.

Where in heaven's name was Ann Maness?

Jens surely must have thought about incinerating the piece of paper on which she was keeping track of their odyssey. But instead she burrowed the notes deeper into her uniform. She was taking an enormous risk, but it was helping to keep her mind active and her spirits alive.

A group of Italian soldiers escorted the Steffa-Abbott group farther into the mountains. As dusk fell, worn-out from the day's strain, they reached another village.

Steffa sought out the village elder, who arranged sleeping quarters and a meal of corn bread and cheese. Abbott and the others continued to question Steffa about the Germans' behavior in Berat. Now that the enemy had their pictures, it would not be good for the Americans, Steffa reiterated.

"For you, bad—if they catch you," Abbott quoted Steffa as saying. "But they don't catch you yet."

"What do you mean 'yet'?" Abbott challenged.

"In war, you do not ever know," came a diffident response that must have sent chills down their spines.

Morale didn't get any better when Steffa shared the sad news that the male lead in the musical they'd seen the night before had been killed by German artillery fire as he tried to defend the village.

"Last night he sings; he is beautiful," Steffa said wistfully.

The Americans may have been touched by Steffa's tribute but couldn't help but wonder how he could know about the singer's fate—yet seemed powerless to get news about the other Americans.

Abbott remembered Hasan's warning that life was cheap in Albania and that practically everyone had a price.

Was Steffa leading them to freedom? Or was he being bribed to lead them into a trap?

The deeper they got into the mountains, the more suspicious they became. Abbott's group had grown jaded about Steffa, questioning the veracity of much of what he was saying.

Jens's group, meanwhile, was following a teenager who couldn't communicate where he was going and may or may not have understood that they needed to reunite with a separate group of Americans.

Uppermost in their minds as they glanced backward was that the Germans were no doubt passing out their pictures to BK guerrillas—and placing a bounty on their heads.

It had been a nightmarish week. By now, they reckoned, those unspeakable telegrams were being sent to their families.

Economist John Kenneth Galbraith, a Roosevelt administration analyst during the war, studied the efficacy of Allied intelligence operations against Hitler. His postwar assessment gave high marks to the combined British-American efforts in Eastern Europe.

"The Americans, as did their British counterparts," Galbraith wrote, "helped to hold in the Balkans German divisions desperately needed elsewhere for combat, and thus made their own contribution to victory."

The grit of the Albanian people also mightily contributed. As noted by the SOE in its midwar analysis, because Mussolini conquered the country before the war officially started, "Albania was the first country to meet the challenge of the New Order with guerrilla resistance in the mountains." That resistance was scattered at first but, after 1941, thanks to the single-minded persistence of Hoxha and his underlings, quickly grew in strength.

Indeed, it's ironic that the first successful Communist insurrections since 1917 were abetted by Great Britain and the United States, the very countries that had sent troops into Russia in a fruitless attempt to reverse the Leninist uprising.

For the first three years of World War II, the machinations of Yugoslavia's Communist Partisans and their rivals, the monarchist Chetniks, were largely ignored by London and, later, Washington. It wasn't until the Allies mopped up North Africa and began heading north in the Mediterranean theater in the summer of 1943 that Britain's SOE and America's OSS began focusing on the byzantine Balkan resistance movement.

"A [Balkan] war that had been shrouded in obscurity and

confusion began to loom larger in the thinking of Allied strategists," observes contemporary British historian Roderick Bailey. The Allies could no longer ignore the savagery of the Nazi treatment of the Balkans, especially since intelligence reports confirmed that Hitler had ordered SS head Heinrich Himmler to liquidate any threat to Axis control.

One of the first Balkan "freedom fighters" known to Churchill and FDR was Yugoslav colonel Draza Mihailovic, an ardent monarchist whose Chetniks were determined to restore to the throne in Belgrade the deposed King Peter. The Allies were initially inclined to support Mihailovic; as time wore on, however, he seemed more concerned about gaining revenge against his internal foes than in fighting the Axis.

Mihailovic had been so beloved in certain Allied quarters that he was the hero of a documentary film that had gone into production in 1942. But by the time the film premiered in London a year later, Mihailovic had fallen out of favor with the Brits and, to a lesser extent, with the Yanks. The title of the movie was changed to *Undercover* and revamped to spotlight Marshal Tito's Partisans. Mihailovic was furious that the Allies were aiding his archenemy; he began openly collaborating with Rome and, by extension, Berlin.

"Now is the time to beat the Communists to their knees, if we act wisely," Mihailovic told his enablers.

The Axis powers, too, began recognizing the potency of the Partisan movement. On January 20, 1943, Hitler and Mussolini unleashed Fall Weiss (Operation White), throwing eight divisions and various Croat units, as well as the Luftwaffe, at Yugoslav Partisans and those villagers harboring them. Tito managed to slip the noose, despite the albatross of forty thousand refugees, many of them barefoot and hungry, clinging to his army.

Under siege from Fascists and Chetniks, Tito begged Moscow for help, but his entreaties went unheeded. It turned out he didn't need Russia's intervention. Tito's masterful escape across a wrecked railroad bridge on the Neretva River with the Germans and Italians in hot pursuit, punctuated by a surprise attack that pummeled the Chetniks, was the stuff of legend. The heavily bearded Chetniks began begging villagers for razors so they could blend in with the populace to avoid annihilation. It didn't work. Tito was merciless.

By late winter of 1943, the Brits, impressed with Tito's Houdini-like grit, had established an SOE mission in Yugoslavia, strengthening their commitment to the Partisans and rupturing ties with Mihailovic. The Americans, however, were skittish about backing the Communists and continued to support Mihailovic, angering Tito, Hoxha, and SOE, Jon Naar recalls.

The frustrated German high command now vowed, once and for all, to crush Tito and his proletarian followers. In early spring of 1943, Hitler launched Fall Weiss's successor, Fall Schwarz (Operation Black). Nearly a hundred and twenty thousand Axis troops and their mercenaries began chasing Tito through Yugoslav mountains and caves. Tito lost some sixty-five hundred men of his nineteen thousand–strong force, but again slipped away.

The marshal had nine lives. A year later, on May 7, 1944, Tito's fifty-second birthday, the frustrated Germans parachuted in a crack SS unit to hunt him down. The paratroopers soon had Tito surrounded in a forest. Again it looked like he was a goner. But he and his men made their way to an old train that chugged out of the woods as German bullets clanged off its side.

"[Tito] was always encircled," Himmler snapped at war's end. "And the man found a way out every time."

Brigadier General Fitzroy Maclean, a thirty-two-year-old Tory MP, an intimate of Churchill's, and a onetime Moscow-based envoy, became the head of SOE's forces in Yugoslavia.

Maclean's admiration for Tito was instrumental in persuading the Allies to end their aid to Mihailovic.

The Moscow veteran had an ear attuned to Stalinist propaganda. Maclean saw "the familiar Communist jargon on everyone's lips, the same old Party slogans scrawled on every wall and a red star, [and] hammer and sickle on the cap badges."

In late November 1943, some two weeks after the crashlanding of the C-53 in Albania, Maclean managed to secure a one-on-one meeting with Churchill in the aftermath of the first Cairo conference with FDR and Chiang Kai-shek. Churchill was lying in bed smoking a cigar and sipping brandy in a Mena House Hotel suite within sight of the pyramids. Maclean warned Churchill that in a postwar Yugoslavia, Tito would "inevitably" establish a Communist government.

Ever the Machiavellian, the prime minister queried Maclean: "Do you intend to make Yugoslavia your home after the war?"

"No, sir," Maclean responded.

"Neither do I," came the PM's biting retort.

Churchill and—to a lesser degree—FDR shared the same priority: to keep the Russian army and Balkan Partisans killing Germans, no matter how distasteful their politics.

FDR at one point wanted to put OSS head Donovan on the ground in Yugoslavia to try to reconcile the differences between Mihailovic and Tito. Churchill, apoplectic at the thought of Wild Bill mucking up the SOE's handiwork, talked FDR out of it.

Lieutenant Colonel Lynn M. Farish, an OSS operative stationed in Yugoslavia, did a report on the Balkans' mystifying intramural discord. Farish was addressing Yugoslavia, but he might as well have been referring to Albania. Donovan shared Farish's analysis with FDR.

"The situation has from the beginning been terribly confusing, and almost beyond the comprehension of an impartial outside observer," Farish's dispatch began.

"The deep-rooted causes of the internecine strife are contained in racial, religious, and political disputation which are so long standing that the people themselves don't understand them. . . . Their first enemy is the other, with the Germans second. . . . It is useless now to endeavor to decide which side first did wrong." Farish, a fine intelligence officer, was killed in a plane mishap later in the war.

Into the Balkans' miasma of intrigue in April 1943 parachuted four specially trained SOE operatives: Major Billy McLean, Captain David Smiley, Lieutenant Gavan "Garry" Duffy, a demolition expert, and Corporal Willie Williamson, a radio operator who'd been trained by the Black Watch, the elite Scottish Highlander regiment. Smiley, a member of the famed Household Cavalry, had served in Syria, North Africa, Abyssinia, and Eritrea before being assigned to Albania.

"Reserved in manner, economical in speech, [Smiley] had a shrewd insight and quiet self-confidence which enabled him to make up his mind quickly and speak with with a directeness that compelled attention without giving offense," observed his SOE colleague Peter Kemp.

Unlike many of his comrades, Garry Duffy did not hail from a privileged background with a public school pedigree from Eton or Sandhurst, the British equivalent of West Point. Originally from Dublin, the Duffys immigrated to Leeds in Yorkshire when Garry's father couldn't find work in the Old Sod. Schooling for young Duffy ended when he left St. Mary's Elementary at age fourteen. His dad died young, so Duffy was needed to help his mother and brothers make ends meet. Before the war broke out, he spent three years working construction in Yorkshire.

His mechanical aptitude earned him a coveted spot with the Royal Engineers. Duffy the engineer became one of Monty's Rats as a member of the Eighth Army's 7th Armoured Division in the North African desert. His bomb-making and mine-laying skills, which Kemp described as "uncanny," caught the attention of SOE once the Afrika Korps was put on the run in early 1943. Soon Duffy was being taught the art of sabotage behind enemy lines.

Duffy was tall and wiry, with dark brown eyes that flashed when angry, a sallow face, thick eyebrows, and an on-again, off-again mustache that tended to droop when its owner was subsisting in the bush. He could never disguise his disdain for foreigners of all stripes, Smiley recalled.

"[Duffy] would have agreed that 'all niggers began at Calais,'" Smiley wrote in his memoir, *Albanian Assignment*. "He had no love of Greeks or Albanians, or for their food or their habits, but he was a brave and resourceful officer who proved his value on the spot." Duffy's contempt for Balkan food was a source of great amusement. "He was always saying 'I can't eat this muck,' and 'Oh! For a steak and kidney pie, or roast beef and Yorkshire pudding,'" Smiley wrote.

Duffy's unfamiliarity with French nearly cost him his life. Soon after parachuting into the Balkans, Smiley was leading a nocturnal

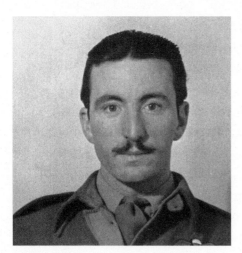

mine-laying raid near the Greek-Albanian border with native fighters who knew more French than English. They were almost finished when an enemy plane suddenly flew overhead, dropping a string of bombs. Smiley hollered, *en français*, for everyone to clear out. Duffy, intent on setting his explosives, didn't understand the imminent danger. Luckily, the bombs missed him.

A Royal Engineer, Lieutenant Garry Duffy was an SOE demolitions saboteur.

No amount of training could prepare the BLOs for the Balkans' crudities. Williamson remembered having to relieve himself outside an Orthodox monastery. In mid-squat, he was appalled to watch an old woman draped in black sidle up next to him, lift up her skirt, shove down her knickers, and "blethered twenty to the dozen. And I thought, 'Good Heavens, I've landed in the Middle Ages.'"

McLean, Smiley, Duffy, and Williamson began their sojourn in northern Greece that spring, but per orders, eventually worked their way northwest into Albania. Following instructions from their superiors in Cairo, they hooked up with Hoxha's LNC. On the night of May 16, 1943, they witnessed Hoxha's Partisans carry out a cheeky assault against an Italian garrison in the southern Albanian village of Leskovik. Badly outnumbered, the Partisans still managed to kill twenty enemy soldiers and destroy or capture twelve trucks and two armored cars. Smiley and McLean, both right-wing Tories, loathed everything for which the Communists stood, but came away from the Leskovik attack impressed by the willingness of Hoxha's followers to take the fight directly to the enemy.

"They [Hoxha's fighters] never relax," the SOE's analysis of the Leskovik raid recounted. "The Italians had to summon aircraft to their rescue, beside a battalion of troops from Korçë; on their return to Korçë, these reinforcements were ambushed at a wooded point on the road and suffered casualties." A "fortnight earlier," the report said, the Partisans had pulled off a similarly nasty raid on an enemy garrison near Derven, inflicting heavy casualties and forcing the Italians to call in another batch of reinforcements.

Soon the BLOs had established a base at Shtylle, some ten miles east of the Italian fort at Leskovik. In touch with Cairo almost every night through their B2 wireless sets, the Shtylle mission began receiving steady parachute drops of food, ammunition, explosive materials, weaponry, and other supplies.

Duffy the demolitionist could make a bomb out of practically anything. He began teaching Partisans how to blow up roads and enemy installations, which his charges began doing with relish throughout southern and central Albania. The BLOs also taught the Partisans how to decapitate enemy motorcyclists by stretching an imperceptible wire across a road. Each time a motorcycle driver was killed, the Germans would exact vengeance on nearby villagers, often assassinating a dozen or more innocent Albanians. The SOE knew the arithmetic was vicious, but its operatives continued to pick off enemy couriers.

On September 3, 1943, acting on a tip, a detachment of Italian soldiers, apparently oblivious to the fact that Italy's new government was on the verge of capitulating to the Allies, launched an attack on the British mission in Shtylle. The Italian attack came out of the blue; it looked as if the Brits and their Partisan allies would be overrun. But Duffy sneaked out and set off an explosive in the middle of the Italian line, precipitating a pell-mell retreat.

He was, as the American refugees soon learned, indomitable.

Many of the SOE officers in the Mediterranean theater were Tories along the lines of Smiley and McLean—conservatives who preferred the restoration of the monarchy to the anarchy of a people's rebellion.

Not so Jon Naar. Leonard John (he deleted the "h" early in life because he thought it gave his name a neater graphic look) Naar had a background almost as elite as that of the archetypal SOE officer. He was a graduate of England's prestigious Mill Hill School, where he captained its under-fifteen rugby team and served in its Officer Training Corps. At age sixteen, he became a Francophone while assuming his studies at the Sorbonne in Paris. While still in his early teens, he broke away from his father's Tory politics to become a Labour devotee, supporting Mahatma Gandhi's bid for Indian independence and other acts of colonial insubordination. Young Naar's convictions weren't theoretical; he took them to the streets. While in his last year at Mill Hill, he fought in the East End against the Blackshirts of Sir Oswald Mosley's British Union of Fascists and their bullyboys in the London police. When he got home he fibbed and told his mother that his facial bruises had come from playing rugby.

Not many Jews of Naar's generation matriculated at Mill Hill. The son of a twice-decorated Great War hero who became the first Jewish mayor of Hendon, Naar at first endured obligatory "Jew boy" beatings at school. But because he was more athletic than most of his Christian tormentors, eventually they left him alone.

His time at the Sorbonne solidified his left-wing leanings. It coincided with the Spanish Civil War and the diabolical cabal of Generalissimo Francisco Franco, Adolf Hitler, and Benito Mussolini. When Paris's International Exposition for Art and Technology in Modern Life opened in 1937, Naar, by then a serious devotee of painting and photography, guided tourists through the pavilion that featured Pablo Picasso's *Guernica*. Naar watched thousands of visitors become mesmerized by the master's indictment of Fascist slaughter.

Disillusioned by what he viewed as Stalin's betrayal of the Spanish Republican cause, Naar returned to London in late 1937 after studying German at the University of Vienna. As war approached, his fluency in French and German made him an alluring candidate for MI6, the British intelligence service.

As he trained in London for his commission in the Royal Artillery, he survived the Luftwaffe's brutal bombing raids during the Blitz. His first undercover assignment was in Lebanon, where he assumed the identity of a Swiss journalist named "Jean Bernard." He was tasked at Churchill's personal direction in late May of 1941 with finding out whether the Vichy French would resist an invasion—the PM termed it a "liberation"—by Australian forces then in northern Palestine. Naar confirmed that the local Vichy supporters would indeed resist being "freed." Back in uniform, Naar was appointed political adviser to the commander of the Australian 7th Division during the six weeks of fighting that ensued. After helping to negotiate the cease-fire with the Vichy French, Naar spent seven months tracking down Nazi agents in Lebanon, Syria, and Palestine.

In October of 1942, Naar got additional combat experience commanding an Eighth Army ack-ack unit during the Second Battle of El Alamein. One night he was sent behind enemy lines to pinpoint cleverly camouflaged Afrika Korps supply dumps.

Later that fall, he joined the staff of the British Intelligence Training School at Helwan, Cairo. He was slated to become part of an underground unit that would burrow itself into the Egyptian capital once the city fell to Rommel's Afrika Korps, which fortunately never came to pass. In mid-1943, he received orders to report to SOE's Cairo headquarters in the Rustem Building, about three miles away. There Major Philip Leake, wearing a uniform with the insignia of the Intelligence Corps, pointed to a topographical map that defined boundaries without identifying the countries by name.

"Know where this is?" Leake challenged Naar as he gestured toward a small territory along the Adriatic. Naar, who'd won Mill Hill's geography prize, knew it wasn't Greece or Turkey. By process of elimination, he arrived at Albania and volunteered as much.

"Well-done, Lieutenant," the onetime headmaster intoned in the inimitable cadence of an uppercrust Brit. "We are looking for an IO [intelligence officer] for Albania," he said. "Interested?"

Leake explained that the more enemy troops that SOE and the native resistance could keep occupied in the Balkans and away from the Italian or Russian fronts, the better.

A few days later, still knowing virtually nothing about Albania, Naar was installed in the SOE section dubbed B8 (the "B" stood for Balkans). The job came with a promotion to captain, a welcome coup for the ambitious twenty-three-year-old.

Captain Naar's responsibility was to keep Leake and others in the need to know au courant with the activities of the BLOs, their allies, and their adversaries throughout the B8 region, including the important job of briefing the BLOs before they went in and debriefing them after they came out. Each BLO in the field was equipped with a B2 set; they were expected to check in with Cairo on a regular basis, but that, Naar recalls, was usually more hope than reality.

Naar had been a football (soccer) buff as a kid, rooting for Arsenal, the north London squad affectionately known as "the Gunners." Arsenal's radio announcers had devised a unique numbering system to describe the positioning of players on what they called "the grid." Naar adapted a similar approach to keeping track of machinations in the southern Balkans. He found an outsize tourist map of Albania in a Cairo bookstore, tacked it to a wall near his desk, and divided it into east–west and north–south partitions. He marked the location of Albania's combatants with multicolored pins: white for the BLOs, black for the Germans and Zogists, green for the Italians, red for the Partisans, and blue for the Ballists. Locations of subjects could be identified by matching the vertical lines of the grid running alphabetically from west to east with the horizontal lines running from south to north. Thus Elbasan might have read "M18."

To shorten radio signals and to save map space, Naar used abbreviations, such as "Alb" for Albania, "bods" for bodies (live ones dropped or boated into "Alb"), "Huns" for Germans, "Jugs" for Jugoslavs, and "pzns" for Partisans. His map got crowded in November 1943 when word reached Cairo about the American plane crash-landing in B8's territory. Each night Naar had to move his pins to account for the sometimes conflicting information he was getting about the whereabouts of the nurses, medics, and airmen and the BLOs trying to find them.

The pin representing Lieutenant Garry Duffy had for five weeks that fall been positioned in the wilds of south-central Albania. Now the pin inched closer to Krushove as Duffy, eager to be the first to "find" the nurses, hiked toward SOE's southern Albanian hideaway.

The morning of November 16, twenty-four hours after the German raid on Berat, the Abbott group woke up scared and agitated. None of them had slept much.

Steffa had told them the night before that the other group was just an hour or so behind. Now he was saying the other contingent was three or four hours away.

As they waited around that morning they couldn't help but notice that Steffa was still showing them off to villagers, perpetuating the falsehood that they were an Allied invasion force to make himself look more important. They felt like they were a "traveling circus," Abbott remembered. Given their experience in Berat, it was beginning to rankle.

They also began wondering whether they wouldn't be better off heading toward Albania's border with Greece. Surely there were more Allied operatives in Greece than in these mountains. The Brits could be anyplace in Albania.

The Americans huddled and agreed that they had to ask Steffa pointed questions. Since the nurses were officers and had seniority, two city-bred women, Tooie Dawson from Pittsburgh and Ann Markowitz from Chicago, were designated point people.

Lieutenant Dawson told Steffa they wanted to wait until the other group caught up before shoving off that day. Steffa shook his head, smirking that no, that would be foolish—the other group would not be coming this way.

How did he know that? Dawson challenged. What about heading back down the mountain and trying to meet the other group halfway?

Again, Steffa was dismissive, saying that would be more foolish than staying put.

Markowitz, without being confrontational, reminded Steffa of their real objective: to find the British officers. Yes, Steffa said, he would take them to the British—but he didn't know where they were.

What about getting to Greece? they asked. That, too, would be foolish, came the reply.

"It was like trying to pin down a breeze with a thumbtack," Abbott would remember.

The morning of the sixteenth did not go well for Jens's group, either. Soon after dawn, the Americans watched two fierce-looking LNC fighters pull Johnny into an animated conversation. The teenager seemed alarmed as he told their group they would need to leave right away.

Within minutes, they were out on the trail. Once they cleared the village, they asked Johnny about the other American group. Johnny seemed confused but then grinned and pointed forward, as if to say, "Follow me." They exchanged troubled looks; Johnny wasn't exactly inspiring confidence. The group was beginning to miss Hasan's steady hand and grasp of English.

Each time they walked past a settlement, they'd hector Johnny about checking whether anyone had seen the other Americans. Heads would shake, Johnny would shrug, and again they'd push forward.

Later that morning they bumped into a horde of a hundred or more Italian soldiers. The *soldati*, who at that point had been roaming the hills for nine weeks, were incredulous to find Americans—especially American women!—in Albania. No fools, the Italians decided to trail them, figuring that the Americans were far likelier to be "rescued" or fed than they were; by their glomming on to the newcomers, maybe something good might happen.

They made quite a "little army," Jens recalled, as they climbed the next hill. Knowing that German planes would not hesitate to strafe their former Axis partners—many of whom, Luftwaffe pilots knew, were now in cahoots with the Partisans—the Americans found themselves nervous walking with so many uniformed nomads.

As they neared the summit, they had to negotiate a slope filled with slate rock. The sharp stone sliced up their fingers and bruised their feet and ankles as they slid backward. Jens glanced behind her and realized that the Italians had disappeared. She wondered whether they knew something she didn't.

A series of rifle shots suddenly rang out. Jens swore a bullet whizzed by her head. Everyone hit the stony dirt. They were paralyzed, not moving a muscle for what seemed forever.

Eventually, Baggs peeked his head up and whispered that he'd spotted a shack at the top of the ridge. Everyone should stay low and move toward it, he ordered. Crawling over the rocks proved painful. After a few seconds, several members of the party took a chance by standing up halfway. More shots rang out. Everyone plunged back down headfirst. It took another fifteen minutes for them to wriggle to the shack, bloodying their hands and knees.

When they got to the door, a sergeant leaned forward to push it open, exposing himself to fire. Fortunately, their assailants—whoever they were—were lousy shots. The bullets didn't even hit the shack.

The hut had but one window, which happened to look out over

the ridge from which the shots were coming. As they stumbled into the dwelling, Baggs yelled for everyone to stay down and away from the opening.

Johnny and the other guides agreed it was the BK doing the shooting. The only weapon the Americans had at that point was Baggs's sidearm, plus the few rifles carried by Johnny and the other guides.

They prayed the Barleys wouldn't make a dash toward the house, because there was little chance the Americans and their Partisan friends could fight them off.

A wounded Partisan suddenly appeared in the doorway, propped up by two comrades. The man had a badly lacerated leg. Jens and the other nurses ripped off his pant leg and cleaned the wound. He was in such pain that he'd bitten through his lower lip. Lieutenant Tacina applied a pressure bandage, dressed his leg wound with sulfa powder, and gave him a shot of morphine.

Two more injured guerrillas materialized; Tassy, Jens, and the others cleaned their wounds, too, then sat against the shack's wall to catch their breath.

It was already past two o'clock. The firing had stopped. Maybe the Ballist attackers had left; maybe not. They couldn't take the chance. Everyone agreed with Johnny that they had to slip away before darkness fell; otherwise they'd have no way to defend themselves.

Their plan was to make a run for a stone wall that led to a hillside path and toward the next Partisan stronghold. Three sergeants attempted a trial run, digging toward the wall, but quickly dived back into the hut when bullets splattered the ground in front of them.

Another fifteen minutes elapsed. A young Albanian came into the shack to confer with Johnny. Johnny gestured that it was okay for them to leave.

Not taking undue risks, everyone ducked as they ran along the stone wall and up the trail to the next village. It was getting closer to the winter solstice; darkness was beginning to descend quicker. It was several hours past sunset when, groping along the trail, fearful of another ambush, they finally arrived at the next safe house.

Johnny had to wake its occupants and whisper into the ear of an older gentleman, who agreed to let the Americans and their protectors into his home. All seventeen Americans tried to sleep in a room that was considerably smaller than the previous night's space. They had neither eaten nor had a sip of water since the day before in Berat.

The Abbott group had it a bit easier. On the morning of the seventeenth, they encountered an Italian colonel on the trail. He developed an immediate infatuation for Ann Markowitz, offering the lanky Chicagoan anchovies and a shot of his *raki*. The moonshine scalded her throat so badly that she kept fanning herself as they took their leave to resume the march up the mountain. Her pals kidded the birthday girl about the dangers of accepting drinks from strange men.

From a distance that morning the Abbott group spotted an Allied air attack. Puffs of flak could be seen beyond the next range. But they were too far away from the attackers to tell whether the bombers were British or American.

They entered a village called Burgulla about three o'clock that afternoon. Steffa pronounced it satisfactory, saying they'd spend the night. There was a small hospital where they had dinner and where the nurses ended up bunking. As they finished their meal, they watched as a Partisan gunshot victim was brought in for crude treatment. There wasn't enough chloroform to keep the wounded man from screaming.

Three young Albanian women entertained them, dancing and singing songs a cappella. They asked the Americans to respond in kind. At first they demurred, but then Tooie Dawson began trilling the Negro spiritual "Ain't Gonna Grieve My Lord No More." The rest of them chimed in where they could, the old saw's lyrics lost on the Albanians.

Oh, the Deacon went down,
To the cellar to pray,
He found a jug,
And he stayed all day. . . .
You can't get to Heaven on roller skates,
You'll roll right by them pearly gates.
You can't get to Heaven on a rocking chair,
'Cause the Lord don't want no lazybones there.
You can't get to Heaven in a limousine,
'Cause the Lord don't sell no gasoline.

There were no roller skates to be had in Albania. And if they wanted to survive, there'd be no lazybones. "Ain't Gonna Grieve My Lord No More" became a staple, one of the songs they liked to sing along the trail when they weren't worried about Barleys or Germans lurking nearby. Soon they knew every verse.

Just as they retired for the evening in Burgulla, Steffa told them he'd been informed that Jens's group would be arriving at any minute, ten o'clock at the latest. The LNC network, Steffa told them, had spotted the other group that morning in the same village that the Abbott group had visited the previous day.

Tooie and the rest of her chorus were skeptical. Sure enough: Ten o'clock came and went; there was no sign of the others. Dawson, her voice warm from singing the spiritual, used it to confront Steffa.

Where were they? What was causing the delay?

Steffa admitted he didn't know, but reminded them that they were all "friends." Dawson reminded him that they weren't his friends—they were more like his prisoners.

The LNC did not take prisoners, Steffa replied. Abbott quoted Steffa as declaring, "We do not take prisoners unless they are our friends"—another oddly disquieting comment.

There was nothing left to do that evening except hope the others eventually showed up. They rolled some smokes with what little tobacco was available and hoped their fears about Steffa were unfounded.

Back in Sicily, Major Red McKnight and the other members of the 807th MAES who had not boarded Army aircraft 42-68809 maintained a vigil for their missing comrades. McKnight and his left-behind nurses and medics did not know that the C-53 had gone missing until another planeful of 807th personnel arrived in Bari, twenty-four hours after the first plane was supposed to have landed. An indignant British medical officer, staring at a field hospital full of wounded soldiers, wanted to know what the hell had happened to the other group. When the circumstances became apparent a day later, AAF officials officially declared the November 8 party missing, but withheld for some two weeks notification of next of kin.

McKnight never gave up hope that the C-53 had somehow landed somewhere and that his charges were safe. But prospects looked bleak.

Over time, the 807th received replacements for the missing twenty-six. But being a nurse or a medic in a combat zone, even one removed from the front lines, was hazardous duty. One of the Catania nurses perished in a jeep accident and two more in plane wrecks.

The telegrams informing the Albanian castaways' families that their sons and daughters were considered missing in action arrived at homes two days after Thanksgiving, November 27, 1943: day nineteen of the saga.

Jens's group was up before dawn on the eighteenth, thinking an early start could help them gain a couple of hours on the group out ahead and maybe get them closer to a village that could afford to feed them. The climb was even more jagged than it had been the day before. Many in the group, including Jens, were struggling with dysentery; given their food and water deprivation, it was hard for them to keep their minds focused.

It took them three hours to ascend the first peak. They were up so high some of them got dizzy looking down. Soon they came upon a small settlement. Johnny arranged for a meal of corn bread and goat cheese—their first food to speak of since two evenings before in Berat.

They walked twelve hours that day, not reaching the next safe village until after dark. That night they had their first hot meal in three days: rice mixed with white bean stew. They were so exhausted they agreed to sleep in separate houses. Everyone needed rest to get back on the trail first thing the next morning.

Up at dawn, they were already hiking at 0630. Two hours later, they stopped to rest in a village and learned that the other American group had been there two nights earlier. A village elder took Johnny aside for a private conversation.

The Americans looked at Johnny quizzically. What was he trying to tell them? they asked.

Johnny stammered something about the villager believing that Steffa was a bad man, not to be trusted, someone in league with the Germans.

They were stunned, trying to re-create Steffa's actions in and around Berat to see whether they could deduce suspicious behavior.

Why would a German collaborator run the risk of bringing Allied personnel into his home? Why not turn them in before that happened? How could someone selling out Albania speak so movingly of its desire for independence and freedom?

Hoping the man was wrong, they hit the trail again, declining his offer of lunch. They hiked at what Jens called a "breathless" pace for two more hours before coming upon a village known as Dobrusha. Johnny pointed to an unusual-looking building and said it served as a hospital.

Just then the hospital's front door swung open. Ann Markowitz and Jean Rutkowski burst out, yelling, "They're here! They're here!"

The nurses hugged one another, jumping up and down, more relieved than anything.

Their exultation wore off in a few moments when the nurses began counting heads. There were only ten of them. Lytle, Porter, and Maness were still missing.

As they pondered what had happened to their three friends, they compared notes about how they had gotten separated on the hillside outside Berat. They couldn't figure out how they'd lost touch. Steffa came out to shake hands with each member of the arriving seventeen. Jens wondered whether she was imagining it, but Steffa seemed less cocksure than he'd been in Berat.

The nurses in Steffa's group quietly related that he was "peeved" with them for insisting that they stay put at the hospital and not move on to the next village. But they were sure glad they won the argument. Jens and the others in her group decided to hold their tongues about the unsettling things they'd heard about Steffa.

Right now the biggest priority was to figure out what, if anything, they could do about the three missing nurses.

Many of the medics and nurses volunteered to go back to Berat to look for them. But the more they thought that through, the more they realized how pointless it would be. Without Partisan guides, their chances of finding Berat were not good, let alone their chances of surviving the inevitable skirmishes with Barley and German patrols.

There was a long silence until Steffa joined the discussion. Tooie Dawson, unaware at that point of the ugly innuendo the others had heard, apologized to Steffa about questioning his judgment and asked whether he could help them find their friends in Berat.

He would try, he said, but he doubted they could be rescued at the moment, not with the Germans in stern control. Nobody said anything for a minute as they let Steffa's assessment sink in.

Steffa then lifted their spirits by asking whether they wanted to buy a goat and have it slaughtered for their evening meal.

Hell, yes! he was told, as Thrasher doled out the group's pooled currency.

As they waited for the goat to be cooked, they reviewed the blow-by-blow of their respective ordeals, racking their brains on how they managed to get separated, vowing to never let it happen again, and speculating about what Porter, Maness, and Lytle might be facing in Berat.

Their misgivings toward Steffa did not ease that night when they learned that the slaughtered goat didn't have enough meat on its bones to sustain a stew. They were reduced to another meal of rice and corn bread, which induced much bitching. Their bodies craved protein.

Steffa told them that when they got farther along the trail they'd be seeing British officers. They prayed he was right.

CHAPTER 6

SURVIVING THE BLIZZARD ON MOUNT TOMORRIT

The blankets they used in Dobrusha the night of the eighteenth were infested with fleas and lice; Lois McKenzie remembered how reluctant they were to scratch themselves, for fear that they'd offend their hosts.

Itching or no, many of the Americans woke up ill, suffering the effects of altitude sickness, old soldier's disease, and soldiers' guilt over having sloppily—and callously—deserted three compatriots. Every time they thought about what Maness, Lytle, and Porter might be going through, McKenzie and Jensen had to stifle tears. They weren't alone: Abbott, Cruise, and others were choking up, too.

As the crow flies, the group had traveled little more than a dozen miles or so southeast of Berat. But in the past three days they had climbed some of Albania's most forbidding terrain. They were already at three or four thousand feet above sea level. Their torment was just beginning.

There was a stream nearby, most likely the River Përroi, in which the nurses bathed that morning. At least temporarily they could get the worst of the grime off their bodies. But their hair lice would remain unmolested.

Their Dobrusha hosts couldn't afford to spare any breakfast. Food and shelter were at an absolute premium. The hills were full of Barleys. The Germans couldn't be far behind. So as they bathed, the group knew that they'd have no choice but to plunge onward.

But where? And what was the new strategy for getting out of Albania?

When they got back from the stream, Lois McKenzie and Ann Markowitz, the two Chicagoans, led a pointed discussion with Steffa about what he was doing to contact British authorities.

Steffa admitted he didn't know whether word had reached the British officers in Albania about their situation. He further conceded that he wasn't exactly sure where the Brits were. But he repeated that there was a good chance that a British officer could be found in the villages of Derzhezha or Lovdar or Krushove, all located at higher elevations a few miles southeastward.

The group debated next steps. Markie suggested that they send a runner ahead with a note for the Brits detailing their situation. McKenzie stifled her anger, saying she'd been in favor of sending a messenger from the time Hasan first mentioned the Brits ten days before. Lois asked whether anyone had anything to write on. Jens produced a scrap of paper that she apparently hadn't used for her surreptitious note taking.

They decided Thrasher, as lead pilot, should sign a message listing the plane's type, identification number, the date of the crash, and their location, but—lest the runner be captured by the enemy—rendered in vague terms. And Thrasher would sign using only his initials.

Steffa summoned one of his guides and sent him toward Lovdar with the note. There was no guarantee that the runner would get through. And even if he did, it might take several days—maybe weeks—before the Brits could be in a position to help. Despite their desperate predicament, watching the runner take off lessened their gloom.

Johnny, the wunderkind, took his leave at that point, Jens remembered, disappearing as mysteriously as he had surfaced. He said he was returning to his Partisan unit. Unlike Hasan and Steffa, Johnny appeared to have no ulterior motive; he wanted only to follow orders and help comrades in distress. Though he had trouble making himself understood, he had helped the Americans survive Nazi air and tank attacks and a BK ambush. And when they got separated, his gritty élan had helped safely reunite them.

On the evening of Sunday, November 14, Ann Maness, Wilma Lytle, and Helen Porter had been assigned to a comfortable farmhouse on the outskirts of Berat. Their host, Nani Karaja, was in his forties, a kindly man who seemed to be something of a gentleman farmer. His wife, Goni, a native Hungarian, was considerably his junior. She didn't know any English but caught on quickly, Maness remembered, and could make herself understood. The couple's six- or seven-year-old nephew, Koli, was also staying with them, along with the host's mother, a widow always attired in black who was known as "Mama Ollga."

The three nurses slept on pallets in the parlor. To make sure that no light would interrupt their slumber and to keep neighbors from peering in, Mama took extra quilts and covered the windows.

When the fighting erupted before dawn the next morning, their hosts told them that it was too dangerous to go running into the village. So the three Americans stayed put—and never heard a word that morning from or about the rest of the group. A few hours later, they discovered to their horror that a detachment of enemy soldiers had bivouacked across the road on the grounds of a school. They spent hours watching the combatants from behind one of Mama's quilts.

Goni wandered near the schoolyard and came back to report that the soldiers were mainly Hungarian conscripts. Her brother-in-law, who knew enough Hungarian to get by, told the nurses that the soldiers were aware that female strangers were staying in the farmhouse and would come by to investigate.

"He said not to try and hide—or try to talk to them. We couldn't anyway," Maness recalled.

A few hours later two "nice-looking" young men, blond and blue-eyed, wearing beat-up uniforms, came into the house, but more out of curiosity than hostility. The two soldiers stared at the three nurses, then spoke to the hostess in Hungarian. With a perplexed look, one of the soldiers gestured toward the insignia on the nurses' uniforms. Maness replied *"infermiera"*—Italian for "nurse." The soldier nodded.

They left after a few minutes without conducting a search or asking any probing questions. On the way out, they exchanged a few words in Hungarian with the hostess.

"They indicated that we should just stay there, and that she should take care of us and not to let us go outside," Maness recalled.

Were the Hungarian soldiers acting out of compassion, perhaps taking satisfaction in defying their German masters by not taking the nurses captive? Or had their hosts or a Berat resistance leader somehow arranged a rapprochement, with perhaps some currency changing hands, in a quid pro quo for silence? The nurses never found out.

All they knew was that they were consigned to the farmhouse. They stayed housebound, never venturing outside except to go to the bathroom, for nearly four months.

Steffa suggested on the morning of the nineteenth that the group of twenty-seven head toward another mountain hamlet, this one several thousand feet higher. Derzhezha might have decent food and shelter, he figured. And it wasn't likely that the enemy would chase them to such a high altitude.

The trail was dangerous—one switchback after another carved into the side of sheer rock. They stopped constantly to suck air into their lungs. It took two hours of arduous climbing to reach a summit that was less than a thousand feet above Dobrusha.

When they reached the top, they thought they'd see a valley stretched out beneath them. Instead they were shocked to glimpse a series of other mountaintops, one more intimidating than the next. They were in the middle of a chain of mountains known as the Albanian Alps, the jagged crests that surround Mount Tomorrit, the third-highest peak in the country. The elation of reaching the summit quickly gave way to the stark realization that their trek had just begun.

To reach Derzhezha, they had to go down to go up. The hike downward was just as harrowing. After two more grueling hours, they reached a stream that Steffa declared free of typhoid. They drank deeply and filled their canteens.

Now they had to scale the next mountain. Again, they stopped every few minutes to catch their breath. Some were doubled over with nausea, reduced to throwing up or discharging diarrhea a few feet off the trail. They were up so high that when the sun disappeared behind a mountaintop it was like an eclipse. Suddenly they were groping in the dark.

It was pitch-black when they reached Derzhezha. The place was so remote that they could not imagine the enemy giving chase.

Steffa, at the head of the pack, was greeted by two village elders and the obligatory barking dogs. After a conversation that turned heated, the elders agreed that the party could stay one night. With winter approaching, there wasn't enough food to feed the Americans beyond that.

Dinner that night was white bread, a macaroni dish, a little goat cheese, and some honey. Two women from the village entertained them with Tosk singing and dancing.

It had gotten brutally cold and rainy. The nurses again lent their woolen liners to the men for extra warmth. They divvied themselves up among several homes and shivered through a short night.

The next morning, Sunday, November 21, everyone was supposed to rendezvous at a cowshed outside Derzhezha at 0900 sharp to begin that day's hike. But certain members of the party didn't get the word or were struggling so badly with indigestion they couldn't answer the bell.

Most of them blamed excessive amounts of grainy corn bread and a strange diet for their weakened condition. But everything was contributing to their dysentery: stress, hostile bacteria, unhygienic eating habits, a rarefied altitude, and sleep deprivation. Many of them were constantly coughing and wheezing.

It was another enervating morning of hiking down, then up. The air seemed even thinner than it had been the day before. It took hours of back-and-forth groping to negotiate a few hundred feet of altitude.

At one o'clock they stumbled into the village of Leshnija. A welcoming party of elders greeted them with great pomp and circumstance. A meal of goat stew and corn bread was arranged along with the customary local entertainment.

The medics and airmen received a special treat: some tobacco and a pipe, courtesy of a local Orthodox priest. Fingertips and lips that had been "seared," Abbott remembered, from trying to get the last scintilla of tobacco from cigarette butts now enjoyed leisurely tugs on a communal pipe.

When the elders sat down with Steffa for a confidential talk, faces turned long. The Americans knew it wasn't good news. Steffa said the locals had received unsettling reports that Ballists, perhaps even Germans, were heading toward Leshnija. Earlier in the day the village council had sent out a scouting party, which had confirmed that the BK was indeed on the move—and getting closer by the hour. The Americans were incredulous that anyone could have tracked them into such harsh country.

It would not be safe for the Americans to stay there for more than one night, the elders told Steffa. Given the enemy's proximity, the group would have to hide someplace even more remote: the highest habitable ground in Albania. But Steffa said the journey up and around Mount Tomorrit would require special guides; they couldn't navigate the peak by themselves. Conditions would be too nasty; visibility would be next to nothing.

Dinner and sleeping arrangements were spread among several dwellings that night. Abbott remembered eating corn bread, sour goat milk, and onion pie—and becoming so violently ill that he couldn't digest any of it.

It's unclear whether Steffa warned them what they'd be up against in climbing Tomorrit. Neither Abbott nor Jensen recorded a stern pep talk in their memoirs.

They had already gotten under way the next day and were resting at their first stop when Steffa, looking annoyed, approached them. The guides were alarmed that a family's good-luck emblem— a smoothed-out stone thought to have mystical powers—had apparently been pilfered from a home in Leshnija. Steffa vowed they would go no farther until the talisman was produced. After a few seconds, a red-faced Bill Eldridge fished the stone out of his pocket, lamely saying that he didn't realize it was worth anything and had just wanted to take a little keepsake. Regardless of Eldridge's motivation, it was boorish behavior that must have caused the women to bite their lips in anger. One of the guides returned the stone to Leshnija.

The mountain people believed in mythic spirits. An ancient Tosk legend held that Mount Tomorrit had originally been Tomorr, a giant who fought another mythological beast, Shpirag, over a young woman. The two giants ended up slaughtering each other. Shpirag became Mount Shpirag, another massive peak. The young lady, brokenhearted, drowned in her tears, which became the River Osum.

Halfway up Tomorr's visage, the Americans were worried about drowning in their own tears. At 8,136 feet, the summit of Mount Tomorrit was higher than the altitude their C-53 had reached over the Ionian Sea on that fateful morning thirteen days earlier.

An icy drizzle greeted them as they started the climb, followed by unremitting fog and sleet. A death-black cloud soon descended, spewing such heavy snow that it must have felt like Tomorr was dumping it over their heads from on high.

The cloud seemed to get lower and more malevolent, obscuring the slippery trail. It was an almost-total whiteout. Walking in single file, they could barely see the person in front of them, let alone Steffa and his guides out ahead.

It was getting more treacherous by the second. None of them dared look at the precipice just off the trail. It seemed to go straight down. Any slip could prove fatal.

Jens felt her fingers going numb and was desperate to pull off her gloves and rub them to get her blood circulating. She was also scared that she was losing contact with the people in front of her.

Someone touched her shoulder: It was Jim Cruise, the effusive Irishman.

The wind was howling so badly that they had to scream into each other's ears to be heard. Jens bellowed for Cruise to tell the guides to slow down so they could all proceed together. Cruise hollered back that "Gawd willing" that was exactly where he was heading.

He yelled for Jens to pull down his woolen cap so it would cover his forehead. She then screeched for him to tug off her gloves so she could rub her fingers.

Once Jens got her gloves back on, Cruise plunged ahead. The group was strung out along the mountain; it would take him a while to reach the front of the pack.

Trailing Jens and Cruise, Lieutenant Jean Rutkowski was getting more defeatist by the second. Jim Baggs, immediately behind her, kept prodding her forward. Finally Rutkowski lay down on the path and begged Baggs and the rest to go on without her and to let her die in peace.

Baggs pulled her up and bleated into her ear that she had no choice but to put one foot in front of the other and push forward. She did.

Tooie Dawson didn't want to quit. But amid the worst of it, her frozen feet went out from under her; she slipped over the side and began sliding down the mountain. Gilbert Hornsby dived after her, stopped her fall, dug his boots into the snow, and with help from others, including Jens and Lois McKenzie, pulled Dawson back onto the path. Dawson promptly fell again, but this time stayed on the trail. Again, they pulled her up; she was able to trudge forward.

A few minutes later everything came to a halt. There was much fear up and down the line that they'd gotten lost in the blinding snow—that the guides weren't sure where to take them.

Cruise and Abbott worked their way to the front. They got there in time to see Steffa chew out a weary guide. The man apparently was refusing to take the lead.

The Americans couldn't understand what Steffa was yelling, of course, but it was clear that he was threatening the man's life if he didn't immediately cooperate.

"And in Albania, when the patriots say they are going to kill a man, they kill him. The sands run out very quick," Abbott remembered.

Steffa pushed the guide back onto the trail. Onward they lumbered. It was miraculous that no one suffered a broken ankle or a wrenched knee or some other debilitating injury that might have caused the whole group to get stuck on the mountain. It was doubly miraculous that no one save Tooie tumbled off the path.

Had it continued to snow the party may not have made it. But after nearly an hour of apocalyptic storming, the black cloud disappeared. The snow stopped, the wind died down, and the sun broke through—at least enough so that they could half see where they were going.

More dead than alive, they tumbled into the village of Terlioria at around three o'clock, after six hours on the trail. The villagers who came out to greet them were amazed: No Albanian in his right mind would try to conquer Tomorr in a blinding blizzard.

Worried about frostbite and pneumonia, Steffa quickly arranged shelter. Their teeth chattering, they were divided up among five houses. Jens was placed with Elna Schwant and Jean Rutkowski, the nurse who'd wanted to be left behind a few minutes before. A young girl in the home brought out a wooden tub of warm water and motioned that they should stick their feet in it. They dried their soaked clothes near the fire and sat curled up, backs to the hearth, while the family brought out a warm meal. It was heartfelt generosity; the nurses kept nodding their thanks.

At the various houses the meal was the same: mutton stew with chunks of meat and corn bread with some goat's milk. The Albanian women in Jens's home were stunned to see that the nurses were wearing frilly undergarments—not woolen underwear. They made the shivering sign, arms wrapped around their chests, and shook their heads.

At Abbott's house, the medics and airmen stripped down to their undershorts and stomped around the fire pit. To entertain themselves, they picked the lice out of their shorts and flicked them into the flames, applauding each "sizzle and pop," Abbott recalled.

They spent the night and a rest-up morning in Terlioria, never straying far from their respective fires, awaiting further word from Steffa and Thrasher. At about three o'clock that afternoon the pair walked into Abbott's place. The men could tell Thrasher was suppressing good news. He was smiling like the Cheshire cat and didn't use their usual old-soldier salutation: "How'd ya pass?"

Thrasher reached into his pocket and began reading a note he said was from a certain British national. The runner, it seemed, had gotten through after all!

They crowded around the pilot as Thrasher read the missive aloud, which was written in consummately understated British style.

> Sorry to hear of your misfortune. The hospital at Catania has been informed of your whereabouts—wheels are in progress for your swift evacuation to civilization. . . . Since you're heading this way, you may as well come to Lovdar, where I shall plan to meet you on 01 December, or as soon as I receive word that you are there. We can make plans for your evacuation then.
>
> Signed, Smith
> British Forces

Abbott and company began slapping backs and cheering so loudly that their Albanian host rushed into the room, fearful that something was wrong. When Steffa translated, the man "rose magnificently to the occasion," Abbott remembered, and pulled out a bottle of *raki*. They shared slugs, toasting the great news.

Young Paul Allen kept on repeating, "Wheels are in motion," as if in a dream, Abbott remembered.

The reaction was similar at Jens's place, with the nurses linking arms in jubilation.

They began hitting Steffa with questions: How far was Lovdar? How long would it take them to hike there? When could they start?

His answers were: not far; a couple of days, and when the weather cooperated. They stayed in Terlioria for two more days, through Thursday, November 25, which, back home, happened to be Thanksgiving Day.

Steffa, conscious of the image the Americans were projecting to his mountain people, urged the men to shave. It had been two weeks since most of them had used a razor; their beards had gotten scraggly. The men colluded, however, and decided to keep mustaches; some even fashioned goatees. Paul Allen kept his sideburns as lush as a Kentucky colonel's, Abbott recalled.

It was a linear distance of only a few miles, but it would take two to three days to get to Lovdar, Steffa told them. A Partisan leader named Pandee joined Steffa for this stretch of the trek; he appeared to have an exalted position within the LNC and quickly earned the respect of the Americans. It helped that he knew a little English.

The hike to the (unrecorded) hamlet between Terlioria and Lovdar was flatter but still strenuous. Ferocious-looking female guerrillas greeted them as, marching military-style, per Steffa's direction, the Americans entered the village.

Bob Owen, who looked like a matinee idol, winked "Watch this" at his buddies as he tried to make time with a big-boned, dark-eyed brunette. Not knowing any English, she rebuffed his initial advance, causing Owen to reassess.

"The situation appears to call for a shortening of the line, as we say in the Catskills," Abbott remembered Owen responding. Owen rolled a cigarette and offered it to her.

She stood with her back against a tree, languidly dragging on Owen's butt while giving the American men a disdainful once-over. The others badgered Owen to at least try to kiss her. Owen said he'd give it a shot if the others would take her gun away. Instead of a smooch she gave them the clenched-fist salute and vowed death to Fascism.

"*Liri Popullit!*" the men chorused back.

"And so is your old man," Owen stage-whispered, to malicious cackles.

In the winter of 1943–1944, the SOE Albanian mission most weeks had fewer than twenty operatives on the ground—some stationed at Seaview or Sea Elephant, its bases along the Karaburun Peninsula that were hidden in the same Adriatic caverns used by the ancient Greeks. Despite its dearth of personnel, SOE still managed to make a "bloody nuisance" of itself to the Germans and their collaborators in Albania, Jon Naar proudly points out.

From the moment SOE's mission arrived, it had succeeded in giving the Axis forces fits. A few weeks after hiking into Albania from northern Greece in midspring of 1943, David Smiley was so pleased with his outfit's bridge and road demolitions that he radioed his SOE superiors in Cairo for more equipment. He wanted Garry Duffy and his Partisan trainees to have the wherewithal to inflict more damage. Even the wary Hoxha began to see the value of an alliance with the Brits and the Yanks.

"Here for the first time the Partisans opened their eyes to the help that SOE could bring," a midwar SOE report noted. In an unnamed mountain village not far from the Greek border, Smiley and his boss, Billy McLean, now a lieutenant colonel, set up SOE's initial Albanian headquarters "under the broken minaret of a disused mosque."

Their biggest priority was training Hoxha's First Shock Brigade. The BLOs begged Cairo to parachute in arms and ammunition: all that could be spared that spring and summer were 128 rifles, 177 light machine guns, 65 antitank rifles, and 349 Sten guns. "They found, however, the Albanian quick to learn the use of new weapons," the report maintained, "and like all guerrillas, he cherished his own weapons above all his possessions."

Despite their success, SOE's activities were fraught with peril. In January of 1944, a Partisan raid near Biza engineered by Brigadier General Edmund Frank Davies, whose curious nickname was "Trotsky," went sideways. Davies was wounded and captured, eventually taken to a prisoner-of-war camp in Belgrade, then to the Reich's infamous prison in Colditz, Germany. His adjutant, Lieutenant Colonel Arthur Nicholls, escaped the ambush but died of exposure days later after leading the survivors into the mountains.

The offensive tactics McLean and Smiley prescribed for the Partisans were dictated by the enemy's strategic needs. As an SOE report noted, there was "little loot" in Albania for the Third Reich to expropriate. Occupying the southern Balkans made sense for Hitler only if he kept a steady amount of chrome coming from Albania's mines. "[The Reich's] aim, therefore, was to keep their supply routes open: it followed that SOE's aim must be to cut them. Warfare in Albania began as it was to continue to the end, as a war of roads."

A second SOE mission commanded by Captain Victor Smith in Krushove was waging that war of roads in the Korçë area. His job was to harass enemy convoys, disrupt chrome supply routes, and cut off the Reich's tentacles into Greece. But suddenly Smith and his men were given a new task.

Many Albanians admired Woodrow Wilson's advocacy of international law and Balkan freedom, but none more than a former national gas company executive and regional prefect named Tare Shyti. Tare was already the father of four children—on his way to six—when the U.S. transport crash-landed some forty miles northeast of his home outside Vlorë on the Adriatic coast.

Shyti was an anomaly: a prominent Albanian who was neither an LNC nor a BK activist. He detested political extremism, abhorring Fascism as much as he distrusted Communism.

Like many Albanian families, Tare's had been touched by tragedy. His father, Sulo Shyti, who had served as a vice commandant of one of the ten Albanian battalions mustered to fend off an Italian incursion in 1920, was murdered by an Italian collaborator. But in the unsparing tradition of *hakmarrje*, young Tare gained his revenge. At the age of eleven, he killed his father's killer, earning the lifelong respect of Vlorë-area villagers.

His family was well connected along the coast and beyond: Tare was the first cousin and confidant of Hodo Meto, one of Albania's biggest power brokers. Over time, Hodo, a business partner of BK strongman Xheli Çela, became a Balli chieftain, too. But Tare, his grandson Leka Bezhani says, was appalled by the Balli flirtation with Fascism and stayed neutral.

His grandfather was so revered during World War II, says Bezhani, that some two to three hundred people in the Vlorë area took their cues from him, refusing to take up arms for either side. With strong allies in Tirana, Kucovë, and Korçë as well as the Karaburun Peninsula, Tare had a reputation throughout Albania of being a resourceful operator who could get things done. That resourcefulness would soon be tested.

Eager to rendezvous with the British captain, the Americans were up and out on the trail first thing on November 26. Still, many of them were so enfeebled they struggled to maintain a decent pace. When not reduced to relieving themselves in the bush, they spent much of that day's hike excitedly speculating about the Brits' escape strategy. If by plane, it would be difficult to find a landing spot in the mountains. If by boat, that would mean a long march somewhere west or south.

They spent the night in a mountain hamlet so tiny that neither Jens nor Abbott recorded its name. The medics bunked in a leaky loft, huddled under filthy blankets, praying that wherever they were headed the Brits would have decent food and lodging.

The next morning they were gathered outside to resume the push to Lovdar when a gaggle of German fighter planes suddenly zoomed over, distressingly low. The Americans scattered for cover, hoping that they hadn't been spotted and that the presence of enemy planes did not portend bad luck.

Once they were sure the enemy planes were gone, Steffa, Thrasher, and Baggs moved to the head of the column so they could greet the British officer, if indeed Smith was still in Lovdar. Thrasher, in Abbot's recollection, was still wearing his now-filthy flight jacket; Baggs had donned an Albanian "goona" coat, not dissimilar to a woolen mackinaw, for which he had bartered a few days earlier.

The group arrived in Lovdar, a village of eight or nine houses, around noontime. Standing on the street offering cigarettes to Steffa and the pilots was a man wearing a huge smile, a well-tailored military uniform, and the unmistakable cap of His Majesty's army.

He introduced himself as "Captain Smith," and gestured for them to get out of the weather. He ushered them to the town hall, cheerily shaking hands with each American as they entered. Smith was holding a single apple, which he handed to Jean Rutkowski, prompting the other nurses to facetiously cry foul.

The Americans were thrilled that the Lancashireman cut right to the chase. Plans were being drawn up to get them to the Adriatic coast, where a boat would take them to Bari. It would take a long time to hike across the country; with the right preparation and cooperation, however, he was confident that they could make it. But for the next two or three days, Smith stressed, they would stay in Lovdar to rest and recuperate before heading out to SOE's base in nearby Krushove to obtain the necessary supplies via parachute drops. The Americans were amazed that Allied planes could make drops in such challenging conditions.

Smith was surprised to learn that three of the nurses had gotten separated. He was also taken aback to hear that the group had been in Berat when the Germans attacked on November 15. Smith promised that he'd try to get a status report on their missing comrades, then asked each to provide his or her full name, rank, and serial number so he could transmit that information via radio to Cairo, Bari, and Catania.

The British captain gave Thrasher four hundred dollars' worth of gold sovereigns to pay for their lodging and food in Lovdar—emoluments that guaranteed deluxe treatment, at least for the women.

They were divided by gender, split into groups of five, and taken to comfortable homes. Jens's hosts produced a wooden tub with warm water that looked so inviting it elicited gasps from the nurses. The tub was tiny; the women had to sit with their knees tucked up to their chest. Still, the experience was heavenly.

The next day they got to lounge in bed. For breakfast, a young girl named Nadia brought tea and corn bread on trays. She then volunteered to wash their clothes, a luxury in which the nurses reveled.

Conditions weren't quite as cozy for the medics; in fact, they were calling on Thrasher to get his money back. Abbott remembered the lousy food and the smoky fireplace. His hosts were so concerned about their fresh blankets being infected with lice that they wouldn't let their visitors use decent bedding.

On their last evening in Lovdar, the town elders hosted a banquet in their honor. Jens was so sick that the thought of eating made her body ache. Many of the others were also struggling.

The next morning the group was eager to hit the trail. But by the time they assembled at dawn on December 1, many of them felt weaker. Charged up by Smith's escape plan, they were gung ho mentally. But physically they were as wiped out as their shoes. Smith knew it.

He would treat them gingerly on the hike to Krushove. To lighten their load and provide conveyance for the weary, he had rented six mules. The Americans needed them. Bob Owen and Paul Allen were so nauseated that Smith ordered them onto the mules at the beginning of the march. Before long, Bill Eldridge and Lillian Tacina, both suffering from frozen feet, joined them. Each got a dose of codeine. The remaining two mules were weighted down with supplies.

At some point that morning Paul Allen's mule bucked and tossed him into the snow, drawing much laughter, especially when Allen threatened immediate retaliation. But no one laughed when

Ann Kopsco became the fifth member of the party forced to ride. When they finally reached Krushove, Ann was in such bad shape that they had to carry her into British headquarters.

By then they were all "hospital cases," Abbott remembered. But there was no friendly hospital within hiking distance.

Once they got settled in separate quarters, Smith produced heavy woolen socks—several pairs for each. It was "luxury beyond expression," Abbott recalled, even though the socks were lumberjack large. Many of them took to wearing three or more pairs at the same time so they could fit into their oversize British army boots, which soon arrived via parachute drops. When Gertrude Dawson learned that the Brits would be dropping in boots, she volunteered to record everyone's size, not realizing that it would be catch-as-catch-can—and that women's sizes weren't exactly in stock. The nurses quickly adjusted to the exigencies of wearing multiple pairs of socks.

They were so mesmerized by the noisy nighttime parachute drops that they would race out of their houses to watch them unfold. The planes would come roaring in low; everyone instinctively ducked. On their second night in Krushove, the first cargo plane undershot the target; several chutes failed to open. Only about a third of the supplies could be recovered. But the Americans were impressed when a second plane's drop hit right on the money; they eagerly helped scoop up the equipment and provisions.

By Friday, December 3, day three of their stay in Krushove, many of them were so sick that they had trouble getting out of bed. Lois McKenzie, Paula Kanable, and Fran Nelson came by the medics' quarters that afternoon with beef broth and blankets, trying to nurse the men back to health. Their supplies of sulfa were running low; only the worst cases got any medication. Within a day or two, most were feeling at least somewhat better. The Smith-ordered R & R was well-timed.

The last shipment of shoes was dropped on the night of the

fourth, along with instructions to leave as soon as practicable for the Adriatic. Abbott wrote that the British planes "again thundered overhead, huge, black swift-moving shadows against the moonlit sky."

In addition to supplies, the Brits that night parachuted in a half dozen SOE operatives. Most had already served in Albania and were being sent back to conduct special sabotage in and around Korçë.

Abbott and some of the other medics and airmen happened to be within earshot when Smith greeted the SOE men.

"How're things going, sir?" one of the men, still clutching his parachute, asked Smith.

"Lively," Smith responded. "Quite a bit has been all right."

Then Smith coyly added: "And since you've been away we've had ten beautiful American women visiting us."

"Did you say women, sir? American women, sir?" they asked in what Abbott described as amazement.

"Oh, yes! Quite so!" Smith quipped, before chortling that it was "too bad" they'd be leaving soon.

Krushove's cobbler had taken some of their salvageable shoes and tacked pieces of beat-up automobile tire onto the soles. The Americans thought it was yet another example of how the Italians and Germans had bled the country dry, but found out that inserting tire rubber was, in fact, a standard Albanian cobbling technique. Convinced that they would be a big improvement over their old footwear, the nurses were thrilled to lace up British hobnailed field shoes with heavy metal toes and heel plates. But soon they would learn that British boots would fall apart almost as quickly as American-made oxfords.

On one of their first afternoons in Krushove, Captain Smith, his

SOE boss, a major named Palmer, and a lieutenant whom the group hadn't yet seen paid a visit to Jens and the nurses. Palmer exhibited the smooth charm that comes with old money. The women had no way of knowing, but he was one Charles Alan Salier Palmer, the scion of Berkshire-based Huntley & Palmers, a legendary "biscuit" (cookie) maker whose tasty products first appeared in 1822.

After assuring the ladies that his team was hard at work getting the party ready for its push to the sea, Captain Smith introduced the other officer. He was Lieutenant Gavan Bernard Duffy, "Garry" to his friends.

Duffy made a powerful first impression. He had sunburned skin and piercing, no-nonsense eyes. Whether sporting a beret or a pillbox-brimmed overseas cap, Duffy always had them perched, Abbott recalled, at a "jaunty angle." A batch of blackish hair spilled onto thick sideburns.

Even while being introduced to the nurses, he was every inch the soldier, ramrod straight, not long on smiles and chitchat. As the weeks went on, he would occasionally flash a self-conscious grin, especially after the nurses figured out how they could tease him. Abbott said that Duffy exuded an "easy confidence," projecting a "rugged hard-boiled way" of handling whatever Mother Nature and Hitler's Reich threw at him.

When Duffy spoke, it was in the coarse hues of Yorkshire, not the softer-sounding "U" (upper class) dialect that Palmer, Leake, and Naar used to great effect. Duffy not only hadn't gone to the proper public schools; he'd barely gone to school at all. But by the fall of 1943, he had more than proven his worth as an explosives specialist. He and his Partisan mentees were inflicting headaches on the Reich throughout central and southern Albania.

In fact, while the Americans were in Krushove, Duffy and his demolition team were eyeing a nearby German warehouse and a bridge over the River Seman. When the nurses heard that the

Brits had invited the American men to join them in clandestine maneuvers, they were shocked to learn that the warehouse—and with it, a Nazi base—was in Korçë, just ten miles east.

Here were the American castaways, practically next door to an enemy command center, surrounded by saboteurs who were supplied at night by screeching Allied cargo planes. The whole thing defied belief.

Smith casually mentioned that one night he'd thrown a cape over his uniform and slipped down Korçë's main street just to get a feel for the enemy's presence.

Wasn't he a little light-skinned to expose himself that way? the nurses asked.

"Yes, well, I was awfully dirty at the time," Smith said to great laughter.

On Friday, Jens did the arithmetic and figured out it was December 3; she meekly announced it was her twenty-ninth birthday. When Smith and Palmer heard the news, they somehow came up with butter, cream, and sugar and made something resembling ice cream, sticking the concoction in a snowbank to freeze it.

The entire gang arrived that evening to surprise Jens and sing "Happy Birthday." Jens was touched by the gesture, astonished that hard-bitten special ops soliders were tender enough to throw her a party.

As the Brits were leaving, Major Palmer told the Americans they were expecting a big drop that night, perhaps even additional personnel, known in SOE parlance as "bodies." He expressed hope that within a couple of days, once shoes had been cobbled, clothing distributed, and everyone was feeling a bit better, the party could begin moving toward the Adriatic. Everyone was thrilled that after three weeks of wandering the Albanian Alps, they now had a firm objective—and the expertise and accoutrements to get them there.

At about 2100 the Brits shouted for the ladies to come outside—the supply planes were due. Every building in the village was reverberating; it felt like the planes were going to touch down on the rooftops.

The next morning the Brits delighted the Americans by delivering a pile of hobnailed boots, scarves, long johns, caps, and even a hoard of sanitary napkins that Naar had somehow procured. Presenting the gifts to the nurses were Palmer, Smith, and four new men, all tall sergeants wearing the distinctive blue berets of the Coldstream Guards.

"Oh, look, the 'bodies' arrived!" Jens remembered McKenzie teasing as the Brits entered their quarters. With typical British humor, the officers had not bothered to mention to the four newcomers that the stranded Americans they were going to visit were, in fact, females. The sergeants, awestruck, stared at the young women.

Smith volunteered that an American OSS captain, coincidentally named Smith, had already been dispatched from Bari to help lead the party to safety. Captain Lloyd Smith would work his way over Dukati Mountain and try to intercept them in midjourney, then escort them back over the mountain and to Seaview.

Once the Brits departed, Baggs and Thrasher, betraying the lack of judgment that plagued them throughout the odyssey, volunteered that they knew Lloyd Smith from their time in Bari and doubted he had the savvy to find them. Given the group's hairy situation, it was the last message that should have been shared aloud, especially since Smith proved himself more than competent.

There wasn't much time to continue socializing: Duffy was insisting that they get organized. After the group had been holed up in Krushove for nearly a week, Duffy declared that they would shove off on Wednesday, December 8, at 1000 hours. Their immediate objective was the village of Gjergjevicë; from there, they'd keep slogging southwest.

As they gathered to push off, the Americans couldn't help but be taken with Duffy's appearance. He was wearing a red parachutist's beret propped at a sporty angle, a scarf made out of pink parachute silk, a leather cartridge belt, a pair of baggy battle-dress trousers, and boots equipped with metal cleats. Slung across his shoulders was a Sten gun. His hand rested near the barrel.

Duffy was plotting the day's course with his towheaded aide-de-camp and radioman, Sergeant Herbert John Bell, whom the Americans quickly nicknamed "Blondie." Bell, trained by the Royal Corps of Signals, was, like his boss, indefatigable. The native of Islington in north London soon earned the Americans' confidence.

Bell and Duffy were eager to get started; they were irked that their extra mules hadn't arrived.

Jens, observing Garry like all the others, found him "very tight-lipped." Duffy never felt obliged to explain what he was doing or why.

"I never questioned him," Jens remembered. "He was trained—he'd been in the country six or seven months; he exuded competence in my brain. No way did I question him. And I think the fact that the nurses didn't [question him] kept everybody in line. You know, we were officers; they [the medics] were sergeants."

Abbott and the other sergeants thought Duffy was "hard as nails." They admired his physical conditioning, the way Duffy could handle their punishing daily marches without breaking a sweat.

"[Duffy] was always urging us on," Abbott wrote, "always seeming to be in a hurry to get to the next town."

Thrasher and Baggs, the two male American officers, were also given light machine guns, but they were captured Italian models, not as sleek-looking as the one Duffy wielded. Victor

Smith's gold coins finally succeeded in acquiring a half dozen mules and mule drivers. The group was buttressed by Steffa's and Pandee's presence, plus several other armed LNC guerrilla guides.

Duffy called them together and warned that they would be hiking through territory rife with heavily armed Ballists. It was imperative for them to obey his orders. No acting up or backtalk would be tolerated. They would hike at least five to six hours every day, possibly more, depending on circumstances.

The British lieutenant took his position at the head of the column. The entourage bade farewell to the villagers, Palmer, Smith, the Coldstream Guards, and the rest of the SOE Krushove crew. In single file they began marching down the trail.

As November turned to December, Captain Jon Naar, Major Philip Leake, and the other members of the B8 section in Cairo had been getting increasingly barbed orders from their superiors in London to do more to rescue the Americans. But their hands were tied.

Naar kept looking at his grid map, trying to figure out other ways to bring the nurses and medics to safety. Given the harsh weather, the rugged terrain, and the lethal presence of enemy troops and Ballists, he was stymied. Despite the pressure London was getting from Washington, there wasn't a lot more he or SOE could do beyond uniting Lieutenant Duffy with the stranded Yanks—and hoping for the best. It irritated Naar and his SOE comrades that OSS kept inserting itself into the Brits' rescue operation. They were beginning to regard it as an aggravating diversion from SOE's main objective: intensifying resistance pressure on the Reich.

In between keeping his map up-to-date and briefing the BLOs, Naar had to help prepare B8's overview on the Balkans to Prime

Minister Churchill for the Teheran and Cairo summits in late November and early December. During the first Cairo conference (November 22–26), code-named Sextant, which brought FDR and Churchill together with Generalissimo Chiang Kai-shek, Naar was on call, in case the prime minister wanted a briefing on Albania. The request never came, but he got to see Churchill up close.

In the courtyard of the Mena House Hotel overlooking the pyramids, Naar watched Churchill accidentally trigger a fountain's spray by prodding it with his walking stick, dousing himself and others. Sitting next to the water cascade, engaged in deep conversation, the PM made an emphatic point with his cane—and *whoosh*! Naar and his fellow SOE officers were hardly through chuckling over Churchill's slipup when word came of the prime minister's Machiavellian exchange with Fitzroy Maclean over Yugoslavia's future. Churchill's edict was clear: the Balkans' Communist-led forces were to be aided at all costs—and damn the postwar consequences.

To the best of Naar's knowledge, Churchill was never specifically briefed on SOE's efforts to rescue the American nurses and medics trapped in Albania. Nor did the issue appear on any official agenda at either of the Cairo conferences or in Teheran. Given President Roosevelt's impassioned involvement, however, it would be surprising if FDR did not broach the matter in private discussions.

By the late fall of 1943, the rivalry between SOE and OSS had escalated. Given the number of American airmen bailing out in the Balkans and the strategic importance of keeping Hitler nervous about his southern flank, Bill Donovan had been carping for months about wanting a stronger U.S. presence in the region. At the Quebec conference in August 1943, three months before the C-53 got lost over the Ionian and Adriatic, the Brits and the

Americans had agreed in principle that the OSS would establish operations in the eastern Mediterranean. But SOE staunchly resisted the accord. The last thing the Brits wanted was the excitable Donovan encroaching in the Balkans.

Donovan was so miffed that, while the Americans were still marooned in Albania, the OSS chief wrote a blistering letter to British general Maitland "Jumbo" Wilson, the commander of the Mediterranean Theater of Operations, demanding that the Brits drop their obstructionism. Eventually, a compromise was reached; the Brits ended up permitting the Yanks to establish networks in Yugoslavia, Romania, and other places, which proved instrumental in rescuing some three thousand downed Allied airmen over the course of the war. But Albania remained until late in the war, with only a handful of exceptions, the province of the Brits.

FDR's December 12, 1943, shipboard harangue against Naar did not happen by accident. The president knew it would reverberate through the ranks. Roosevelt's pique betrayed a reality that the Brits were only then coming to appreciate: Two years after Pearl Harbor, Washington was asserting primacy in everything, including tactical decision making. FDR wanted America's now-junior partner to know who was calling the shots—even if, as in this episode, those shots were widely off target, Naar notes.

Lieutenant Garry Duffy and his American brood knew nothing of this geopolitical intrigue as they traipsed through the icy hills of southern Albania.

CHAPTER 7

AVERTING A GERMAN AVALANCHE

On the morning of December 8, as Duffy led the group
down the trail, they could see "VF" (for *Vdekje Fashizmit!*) and
"LP" (for *Liri Popullit!*) painted in massive letters on a distant cliff.
Someone had gone to great expense—not to mention peril, since
BK guerrillas were all around—to brandish the LNC's rallying cry.

Duffy's orders were to get the Yanks to Seaview, the SOE's
Adriatic base on the far side of Dukati Mountain, as quickly as he
could. Clinging to mountain trails, the group planned to make the
trek in two stages.

Stage one would be to hike south to SOE major H. W. "Bill"
Tilman's hideout at Shepr; stage two would be a march southwest-
ward to the coast. Along the way they would hopscotch from one
LNC safe house to another. If the path stayed relatively clear and
they made decent time, it would take them, Duffy reckoned, the

better part of a week to get to Shepr, then another week or more to get to the Adriatic.

Abbott and some of the other Americans naturally wanted to watch Duffy in action, so they gravitated toward the point. Duffy was walking purposefully, neither quick nor deliberate, glancing over his shoulder to make sure his brood stayed in line and constantly communicating with the guides he had sent ahead to scout for Ballists and German patrols.

It didn't take long for Duffy to expose a side that the Americans would come to see as bloodthirsty. As they negotiated the trail, Duffy murmured something about being sorry he couldn't witness the "executions."

What executions? Abbott and a couple of other Americans inquired. Duffy explained that his SOE comrades in Krushove had caught, red-handed, the Albanians who had been stealing matériel from off-target parachute drops. The thieves had been handed over to local Partisan leaders for the administration of swift justice.

Not wanting to challenge Duffy in the first minutes of their relationship, no one expressed their misgivings, at least not within Duffy's earshot. But it seemed inhumane to shoot impoverished villagers who were only looking for a little extra food or clothing for themselves and their families. After all, many of those same locals had, at considerable risk, been harboring the Americans and providing critical assistance to the Brits.

The Americans soon learned that Duffy operated with a commando's hardened indifference. Saboteurs like Duffy didn't spend a lot of time contemplating the moral niceties of the fight against Fascism.

Albanian mule drivers, the Americans also observed, had a fascinating technique for keeping their animals from bolting downhill. The drivers would grab onto the mule's tail with both hands and hold on for dear life, their feet braced against the rocky hillside.

Duffy and the Brits had wisely sized up the Americans' situation. They knew that the escapees' weakened condition would require extra mules. Members of the party too sick to walk were ordered to climb atop mules to avoid collapse or dehydration.

It took only an hour for C. B. Thrasher, the group's ranking male officer, to draw Duffy's ire. Having been warned not to bring undue attention to the group with BK guerrillas prowling nearby, Thrasher nevertheless decided a flock of birds flying overhead might make for an appetizing lunch. He cut loose with his burp gun, creating an incredible racket and scattering the flock, but not surprisingly, failing to drop a single bird.

Duffy, startled, came running back through the column. When he learned that Thrasher had been sport hunting, he was irate. He also wasn't happy to discover that certain members of the group had already begun to straggle. While still seething at Thrasher, Duffy sternly ordered ranks closed.

Maybe the pilot had fired the machine gun to impress the ladies or to "test" Duffy. Either way, it was a boneheaded move, especially coming from the group's supposed leader.

After Duffy's tongue-lashing, they resumed their hike. Eventually they stopped for a break in a small settlement called Voskopoje. The village, a resistance stronghold, had been incinerated by the Italians and Germans some weeks before. Survivors of the attack were inhabiting the charred ruins of what had been their homes.

The group could not imagine that anyone in such grim circumstances could afford to part with food or water. But Duffy, no doubt using the gold sovereigns that Palmer and Smith had provided, emerged from one house with a wheel of wheat bread and a chunk of goat cheese, which he divided among the group. Duffy also acquired some bitter native tobacco the Albanians called *duhan*, which the group rolled into smokes.

At Duffy's order, Blondie radioed ahead to an LNC operative and arranged for that night's accommodations. It was bitterly cold; no one in the group objected when Duffy ordered a brisker pace. At about three o'clock they arrived in Gjergjevicë, another village that had been ransacked by the Germans. The food provided by the Muslim town elders was barely edible; the only blankets available were contaminated with lice. They spent a frigid night quivering around smoking fire pits; most were unable to sleep.

The next morning at 0800 Duffy looked everyone in the eye and told them he was going to push them harder. Bill Eldridge had been up much of the night, vomiting. He was suffering the effects of a bad diet on a bleeding ulcer. Duffy ordered Eldridge onto a mule; the nurses kept a wary eye on him.

As they started down the trail, the nineteen-year-old Paul Allen suddenly discovered that his "lucky" parachute cord was missing from his coat pocket. Yelling that he'd dragged the cord "all over this damned country," he wanted to borrow Duffy's tommy gun to go punish whoever had swiped it. At first Duffy gave him a wan smile and gestured for him to get back into the column. When the teenager persisted in his rant, Duffy snarled, swung his gun in Allen's direction, and demanded he get back into line.

They found themselves in a stretch of southern Albania with seemingly "endless folds of wooded mountains," Abbott recalled. The hills weren't as formidable as the ones they had experienced the week before; still, it was an exhausting grind to reach the hamlet of Panerit.

Eldridge struggled with nausea again that night. Jensen, Markowitz, Rutkowski, and Kanable told Duffy it would be best if Eldridge spent the night with them. Their medical supplies had been replenished in Krushove; they gave Eldridge a shot of morphine, removed the liners from their coats and covered him as best they could, then took turns checking on him.

That Saturday evening Lebo and Shumway were assigned to a Panerit home that, as luck would have it, was hosting a wedding reception. The next morning, the two airmen recounted tales of raucous singing, a drunken brawl, a water buffalo dragged into the house for amusement, and at least one gunshot knocking a hole in the ceiling.

Lebo and Shumway were asked whether the bride radiated "any glamour." Funny you should inquire, the two men replied. There were a couple dozen women at the party—but the American duo never did figure out which one was the bride.

One of the medics volunteered that the only "glamour" in Albania belonged to the ten women in their party—and the three back in Berat.

All these years later, it's the inevitable question: Was there any romantic entanglement among the young women and men trapped for two months in wintertime Albania? After all, they hiked, ate, and—sometimes—slept together, often after a few belts of *raki*. It was far from guaranteed, moreover, that they'd survive. Death or capture could come at any instant—the sort of existential uncertainty that might tempt people to throw caution to the wind.

Interviewers over the years put the question to Agnes Jensen, Jim Cruise, and Garry Duffy. All said no, that they were so focused on mere survival that there was neither time nor energy for *l'amour.* It was also too bloody cold, Jon Naar points out.

"Listen, if you'd have been on that trip, you'd have forgotten all about romance," Duffy told the Associated Press (presumably Hal Boyle) in the winter of 1944.

A half century later, Cruise told Peter Lucas, "Oh, no. We were young, sure. But we were tired and hungry and scared most of the time. You have to understand, the Germans were looking for us. They thought we were part of an invasion force. We had to march from village to village. We were dirty. We couldn't wash. We all had lice. We all had dysentery and diarrhea. I felt sorry for the nurses. We had to stop so they could go into the woods to do their business and to pick the lice out of their hair. Believe me, sex was not on our minds."

Nor was sex on the minds of the missing three that winter. Ann Maness, Helen Porter, and Wilma Lytle slept, ate, and sat in the parlor of that farmhouse week after week. They watched the snow pile up outside and the German-Hungarian encampment across the road break up and leave. But the nurses were never bothered by Ballist fighters or enemy soldiers or anyone else, although a fair number of people seemed to know that they were there. Naturally, the nurses worried that a German sympathizer would rat them out or break into the house to drag them away— but it never happened.

The nurses were stuck—but they weren't kept concealed. It's not as if they were relegated to an Anne Frank–like existence in an attic or a basement. They continued to wear their American garb and walked around the house and relieved themselves in the back-yard outhouse.

They were fortunate that their hosts were well connected and had abundant amounts of food, wine, *raki*, and smelly Albanian cigarettes. The nurses didn't know for sure, but they sensed that neighbors were donating food and drink to their host family.

Riven with guilt, the three kept asking to help with chores

around the house—but their offers were declined by Mama Ollga and Goni. The entire time they stayed in the house they were allowed to wash dishes only a couple of times.

They played unending games of two-handed bridge—Lytle's religion forbade her from playing cards—and some games favored by Mama, whose rules remained murky to Porter and Maness. No one argued too vociferously, Maness recalled, but they occasionally would get feisty just to relieve the boredom and keep their blood pressure from dropping too low. They ate so well that Porter later claimed she gained a few pounds.

Albanian men and women, whom the Americans deduced were local leaders, would come to the house every few days, share a few quiet words with Nani, then depart. Nani assured them that their American compatriots had not been killed or captured in the assault on Berat and that plans were afoot to rescue the three of them. But they would have to wait until some of the snow and ice thawed from the mountains before attempting to slip away. There they sat, month after month, never once straying from the farmhouse and its yard.

On the morning of December 10, Eldridge felt well enough to get off the mule. They shoved off at 0830, with Duffy intending to get to the village of Frasheri by day's end. Within minutes, though, they ran into Albanians who reported that enemy troops and Ballist guerrillas were up ahead. Duffy decided to reroute the group to Costomicka, a strong hour's climb up from the River Osum.

Negotiating the river was tricky; with all the rain and snow, the Osum was running swift. Duffy paid a local farmer to borrow two horses—and put two members of the party on each animal. It took repeated crossings and many precious minutes to get everyone to the far (northwestern) side, with Duffy and Blondie nervously scanning the hills for signs of the enemy.

When they got to Costomicka, Duffy had Pandee question the villagers about Ballist activity in the area. The locals were apprehensive; a village less than an hour's hike away had been roughed up by the BK, they said. Costomicka's elders were worried about reprisals for harboring the LNC. The Germans and the Ballists, operating in concert, had been exacting vengeance killings throughout the region. The LNC, meanwhile, had expropriated more than a thousand sheep from the area, which enraged all parties, but especially the Ballists, who needed the food and wool for themselves.

It all sounded so bleak that one of Duffy's interpreter-guides refused to continue. Duffy, hard-hearted though he was, let the guide vanish. Virtually surrounded by hostile forces, stuck in forbidding terrain, with smoldering villages all around, Duffy's little band was already getting depleted. And they'd barely started.

As if morale weren't already shaky enough, the Americans took to heart a rumor they'd heard from villagers that an Allied army had invaded the Albanian coast and was driving inland from Vlorë and Durrës. Thrasher and Baggs, who as officers should have exercised better restraint, became "light-headed" when they heard the gossip. Jim Cruise and Ann Markowitz got so excited that they grabbed each other and jumped up and down. Duffy quickly pronounced it "a lot of damned rot and bally nonsense," but the Americans couldn't help themselves. They were desperate to glom on to good news and immediately began speculating about how and where the troops might arrive.

Only after Duffy, through gritted teeth, agreed the next evening to radio Bari, and confirmed once and for all that no Allied force had invaded Albania, did the Americans finally calm down.

Having had their hopes artificially lifted, they were now devastated, which had been Duffy's trepidation all along.

Duffy's nightmare scenario soon unfolded. Enemy activity was so ubiquitous that the lieutenant felt he had no choice but to have the party traverse Mount Nermerska, at an altitude of eighty-one hundred feet the highest peak in the area, where chances were they wouldn't be followed.

The new route necessitated another river crossing, this time in all likelihood the River Vjosë. Duffy's Partisan pupils (and perhaps Duffy himself) had weeks before destroyed the stream's only reliable span. In retaliation, the Germans had burned the village of Përmet, an LNC hot spot, on the river's opposite bank. Now the only way over the Vjosë was to negotiate a swinging suspension bridge that must have looked like something out of a Saturday matinee feature.

At 0920 that morning, Duffy told them to spread out in groups of four or five; he feared snipers, perhaps even machine gunners, lay hidden in the woods along the river valley. He advised them to move quickly down the path and across the bridge. Pandee and the other guides unloaded the mules and got everyone and everything across without incident, although the shaky bridge made several in the party even queasier than they'd been.

Waiting on the other side was a dilapidated Italian truck (in Duffy's daily wrap-up he referred to it as a "big WOP diesel") that transported the group the final few miles into Përmet. They found themselves the object of adoration again, although on a much smaller scale than the rapture that had greeted them in Berat. A cheering crowd gathered as the truck, gears grinding, pulled into town.

A town elder thrilled them by leading them not to a municipal building for speeches but to a barroom for some *raki*. Duffy's gold also produced a big basket of grapes and cheese. Plus enough *duhan* to roll cigarettes.

It was an eerie experience, since the Germans had eviscerated the village a few days before; many of the dwellings had been burned to the ground. The people of Përmet didn't have enough food to feed themselves, yet here they were not only sharing what little they had, but throwing a party in honor of their American allies.

Duffy had hoped to use a British-installed telephone circuit to contact the SOE hideaway at Shepr on the far side of Mount Nermerska—but the line had been severed, presumably by the enemy. Duffy had to communicate their plans through guide-messengers and by radioing SOE regional headquarters, which was in the process of being transferred from Cairo to Bari.

The trail up Nermerska was steep—once they reached higher altitude, they had to rest every couple of hundred yards—but not as arduous as the one they'd scaled on Mount Tomorrit. It was cold and windy that day, but they didn't run into a blinding snowstorm. Many of their shoes, however, even the ones that had been fixed in Krushove, had begun to fall apart. Charles Zeiber's boots were so riddled that he said to hell with them and threw them away, preferring to hike in his stocking feet.

The first two members of the party to reach Nemerska's summit were Tooie Dawson and Paula Kanable, the least likely pair to lead them to the top of anything, Abbott recalled. Dawson and Kanable had by then established a reputation of being slowpokes—with sometimes frosty attitudes to match.

Duffy confirmed in mid-December that the American OSS officer Captain Lloyd Smith had, after several failed attempts, been given a fix on their position and was working his way east.

The Americans, no doubt fueled by the pilots' ill-advised cynicism, asked how confident Duffy was that Smith would be able to find them. As long as Smith's radio functioned and his bosses were able to furnish a decent map and a set of guides, he should be able to find them, Duffy said.

Under pressure from his OSS superiors, who themselves were under pressure from the White House, Smith had tried since December 3 to reach the Albanian coast. But *furtuna* and high waves some five miles off the Albanian shore forced his boat to return to Bari. Two days later he tried again to cross the Strait of Otranto, but was forced to abort his landing when the crew thought they heard enemy patrol boats.

Finally, on December 7, twenty-four hours before Duffy's party shoved off from Krushove, Smith set foot on Albanian soil. His boat dropped him several hundred yards off the shore at Seaview, where he was met by a local Partisan paddling a rowboat. The cave that served as Allied intelligence headquarters was some eight hundred feet above the beach; Smith and his guide used an S-curved trail to get to the cavern. Equipped by SOE, the cave had several bunk beds, a crude stove and fireplace, a weapon and ammunition cache, and a large radio that allowed them to communicate with Bari, Cairo, and beyond.

Smith had grown up wrestling in State College, Pennsylvania, tough enough in his college years to have grappled for the Penn State varsity when not studying agronomy. Bowlegged and stocky, with a scruffy blond beard, he was in some ways the inverse of Garry Duffy.

Like Duffy, though, Smith didn't know a word of Albanian. Unlike Duffy, however, he had only the vaguest sense of the intramural struggles among the LNC, the Ballists, the Legaliteti, and all the rest, and would be completely dependent on the warlords and BK enablers who lived along the Albanian coast. His entire preparation for the Albanian rescue mission consisted of one three-hour session conducted by superiors in Bari.

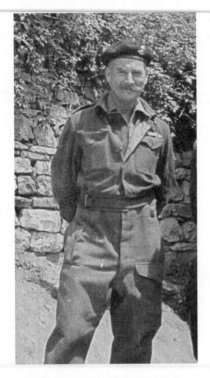

SOE Major Bill Tilman was the British Empire's most renowned prewar mountaineer.

On December 14, after a comparatively easy three-hour hike downhill, the group reached Shepr, a small settlement nestled in a ravine southwest of Nermerska's slope. SOE major Harold William "Bill" Tilman, a mustachioed pipe smoker, was there to greet them. The Americans may not have recognized his name—his public persona was "H.W.," not "Bill"—but Tilman was one of the most celebrated explorers and mountain climbers in the British Empire, if not the world. Seven years earlier, Tilman and another English adventurer reached an altitude of 25,643 feet in scaling a peak in the Himalayas—a world record for summit ascension that would stand until the Mount Everest expeditions of the 1950s.

His military achievements were even more distinguished than his mountain explorations. As a teenage artilleryman, he was awarded two Military Crosses for his World War I heroism along the Somme. In the early days of World War II he survived the debacle at Dunkirk and served as an intelligence officer with the Desert Rats in North Africa. After parachuting behind enemy lines in 1943 to work with Partisans in Albania, Tilman did the same the following year in northern Italy. In toto, he spent an astounding twelve months behind German lines during World War II.

Tilman had plenty of cigarettes, pots of hot tea, and the first Western magazines the Americans had seen since leaving Catania five weeks before. Even better, he had a radio that worked well enough to bring in a jazz station. For the first time in more than a month, the nurses, medics, and airmen could relax and tap their toes to some familiar music.

Baggs, Thrasher, Duffy, and Tilman met for several hours plotting the group's next move. Joining them was Duffy's old running mate, Scotsman Willie Williamson. Duffy asked Tilman whether he could spare Corporal Williamson. Tilman agreed to "lend" the seasoned radioman and saboteur to Duffy.

The rest of the party was thrilled to sit in relative warmth, hum along to the radio, and sip tea. They were in no hurry to get back on the trail.

Alas, ten of the enlisted men were told that there wasn't sufficient space for them in Shepr; they would need to hike to a nearby village, spend the night, then rendezvous in the morning, which happened just after dawn.

The group bade farewell to Tilman and endured a long day on the trail. That night at twilight, things got dicey. As the group approached the village of Gjirokastër, they crossed an airfield that had been abandoned by the Italians. Suddenly Duffy signaled for everyone to hit the dirt, then a moment later ordered them to take cover in a wooded area beyond a fence.

He had spotted in the distance a pair of headlights and feared it was a German truck or staff car. As the others hid, Duffy stayed on the field, crouching, so he could eyeball the vehicle. He watched as the taillights grew dimmer up the next hill, then joined the Americans in the woods.

Was it German? the Americans breathlessly asked.

"Don't know," he answered, which Abbott took to mean "probably yes."

Duffy waited until it was dark before stealthily moving the group up a cobblestone road to Partisan headquarters, which was hidden in a modern-looking schoolhouse. The building seemed deserted from the outside. But they were greeted by an LNC fighter who led them into a room illuminated by two very dim bulbs. The desks and chairs were tiny, meant for elementary school students; the Americans sat awkwardly as Duffy and Pandee discussed the dismal situation with local leaders.

Within a few minutes, the Americans were being escorted to homes for the night. Jens's house was more comfortable than most of the Albanian dwellings she'd visited. It had an indoor toilet, which made taking care of her diarrhea a little less distasteful.

Duffy was downcast, clearly worried about all the enemy pillaging. His fears intensified the next evening when, after hours of hiking in bitter cold, the group arrived at Maskulon, the place that had been their original objective the day before. The village, still smoldering, had been burned to the ground by a German patrol twenty-four hours earlier. Locals, fearing that the Germans would execute them, had run off and were only now returning to their demolished homes. Their livestock and foodstuffs had been stolen. Had, as planned, the Allied-LNC party been in Maskulon the day before, there was a good chance they would have been snuffed on the spot.

Since it was clear the group couldn't stay in Maskulon, a terse Duffy asked for directions to the next "safe" village. As hungry and tired as they all were, they had little choice but to trudge another three and a half hours through the darkness to a settlement called Zhulat. Duffy and Blondie got them housed for the night before disappearing to alert their superiors via radio about the group's precarious status and the enemy's remorseless quest to scorch Albania's earth.

On top of everything else, the Brits' radio was now misbehaving. The Americans, sensing Duffy's exhaustion and frustration, began worrying about him.

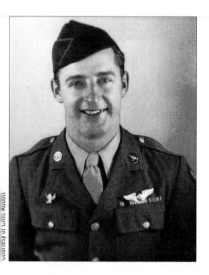

Lawrence Orville Abbott was the pride of Michigan's Muskegon Valley. He was the fourth of five brothers, all of whom served in uniform during World War II. Their father died when Orville was just four.

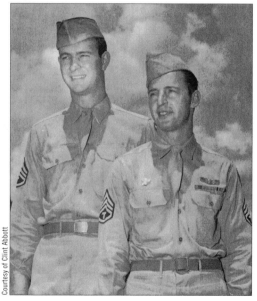

Sergeants Bob Owen (*left*) and Orville Abbott as members of the 805th Medical Air Evacuation Squadron at the AAF Tactical Center in Orlando, Florida, June 1944. Abbott served in two other stateside MAES units upon leaving the 807th after his escape.

British SOE Captain Jon Naar, a northwest Londoner, helped coordinate Allied intelligence operations in Albania. He kept track of the stranded Americans' trek on a large map.

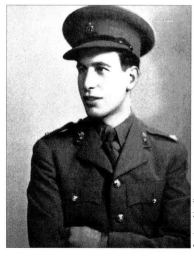

The Americans were greeted as conquering heroes as they entered the walled town of Berat on day five of their ordeal. They spent three days being wined and dined before the Germans attacked, sending them scurrying into the Albanian Alps. Three of the nurses got separated and spent four full months hiding in a Berat farmhouse before finally being rescued.

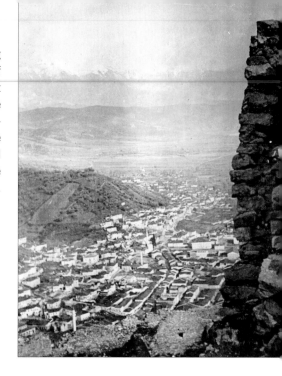

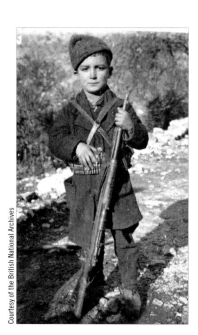

Albanian boys, like this ten-year-old, were pressed into duty to fight the German occupiers. As the war deepened, Partisan leader Enver Hoxha was able to recruit more Albanians to join the crusade to eject the Nazi occupiers. The Partisan army was largely supplied by the British Special Operations Executive.

Albania's Partisan ranks were filled with women, some of them young girls. SOE and OSS operatives were awed by the female soldiers, who fought alongside their male brethren as the Germans were pushed out of Albania in the fall of '44.

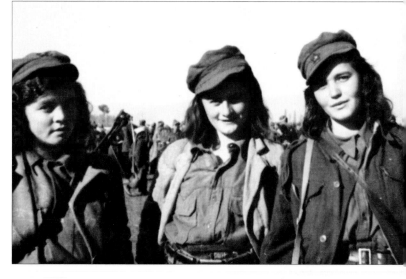

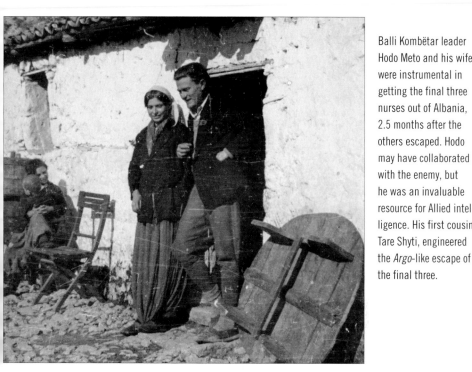

Balli Kombëtar leader Hodo Meto and his wife were instrumental in getting the final three nurses out of Albania, 2.5 months after the others escaped. Hodo may have collaborated with the enemy, but he was an invaluable resource for Allied intelligence. His first cousin, Tare Shyti, engineered the *Argo*-like escape of the final three.

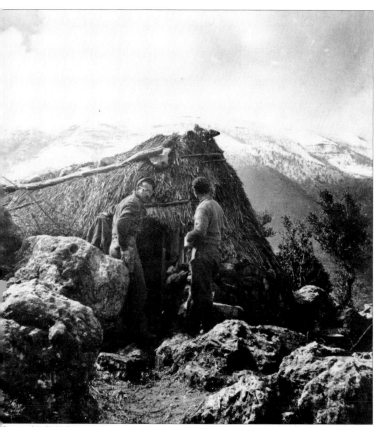

This shepherd's hut in southern Albania was smaller than most of the dwellings in which the American castaways stayed. In many Albanian homes, chickens, goats, and other animals were allowed to roam. One night, near the end of the ordeal, nurse Agnes Jensen's toes were nibbled on by a baby goat.

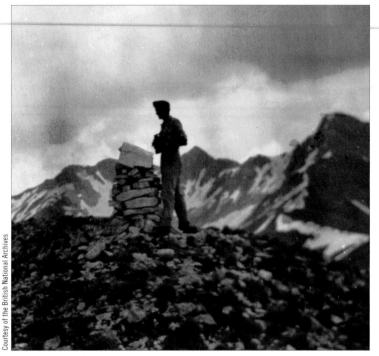

SOE Major (later Lieutenant Colonel) Charles Alan Salier Palmer helped rescue the Americans from hostile guerrillas in the Albanian Alps. The Americans didn't know it, but he was the scion of Britain's largest "biscuit" (cookie) fortune. He survived the war, returning to Huntley & Palmers and British society.

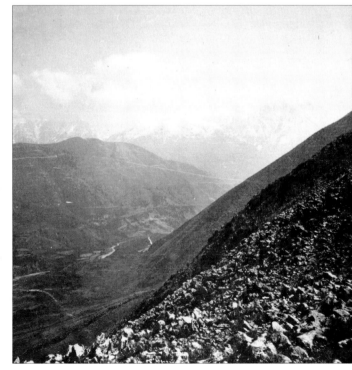

The final mountain that the Americans had to surmount before reaching Seaview and a boat ride to freedom was the Dukati Range. The view of the Adriatic from beyond the snow-filled Dukati Pass was breathtaking. By the time their odyssey was over, they had walked some eight hundred miles up and down Albanian summits and survived three deadly blizzards.

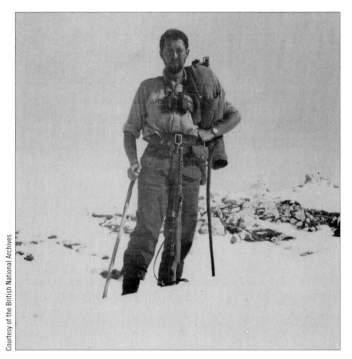

Major Anthony Quayle, the future *Guns of Navarone* star and knighted British thespian, poses at the top of Dukati Pass, February 1944. A German patrol had forced SOE and OSS to temporarily evacuate Seaview and Sea Elephant, their two hideaway coastal bases. Quayle helped plot the escape of the final three nurses.

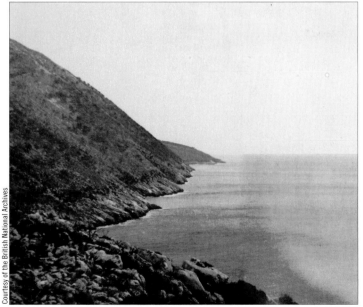

Seaview, SOE's main base on Albania's southwestern coast, served as the embarkation point for the Americans as they were spirited aboard the *Yankee* and taken across the Strait of Otranto to freedom. The SOE and OSS used the same caverns as ancient Greek mariners.

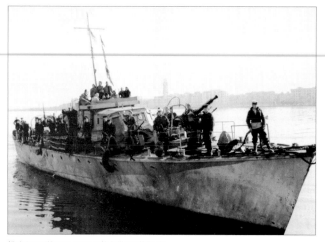

The *Yankee* and its cargo of American escapees arrive in Bari Harbor, Italy, early afternoon, June 9, 1944, after a half-day voyage across the Adriatic from Seaview. The launch was skippered by Hollywood actor Sterling Hayden, an OSS Marine lieutenant. British Lieutenant Garry Duffy (*lower photo*), who spent six harrowing weeks shepherding the party past enemy patrols, is the mustachioed officer wearing the cap.

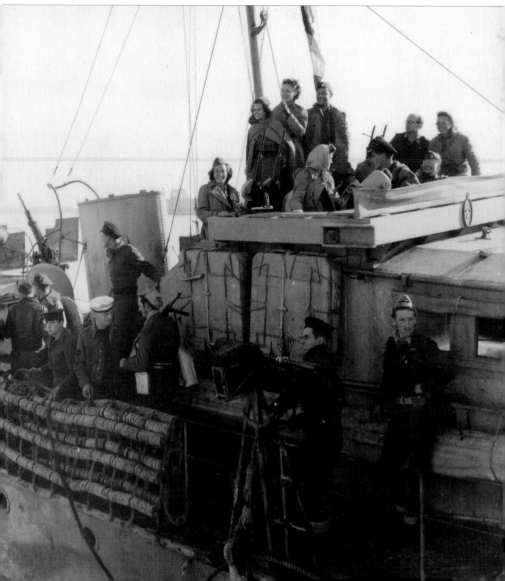

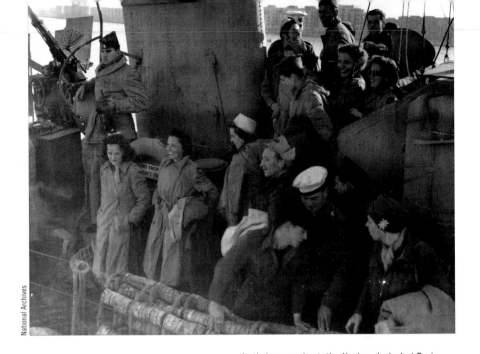

As their rescue boat, the *Yankee*, docked at Bari Harbor, the nurses began to realize their sixty-two-day nightmare was over: (*left to right*) Tassy Tacina, Ann Kopsco, Tooie Dawson (*white cap*), Paula Kanable (*peaked cap*), Ann Markowitz (*in hair wrap obscured by Kanable*), Jean Rutkowski, and (*in sunglasses*) Lois Watson McKenzie.

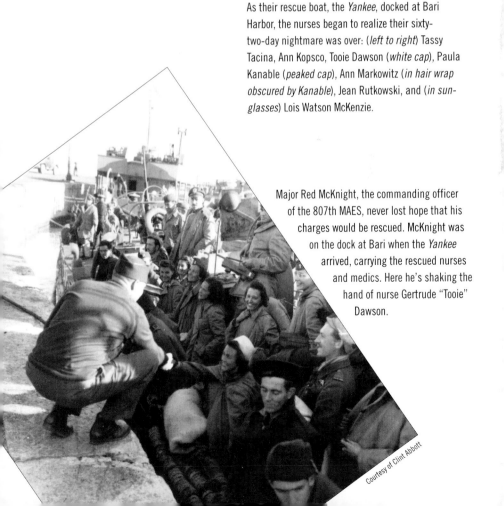

Major Red McKnight, the commanding officer of the 807th MAES, never lost hope that his charges would be rescued. McKnight was on the dock at Bari when the *Yankee* arrived, carrying the rescued nurses and medics. Here he's shaking the hand of nurse Gertrude "Tooie" Dawson.

Just minutes after the rescue boat arrived in Bari on January 9, 1944, British SOE Lieutenant Garry Duffy (*foreground*) posed for 15th USAAF photographers with nurse-lieutenants Jean Rutkowski (*left*) and Ann Kopsco.

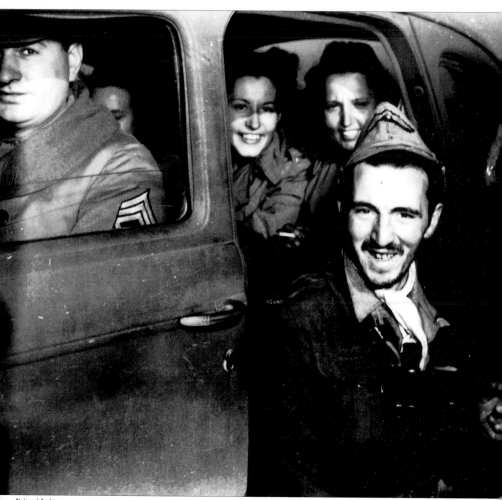

A freshly shaved Duffy beams as Lillian Tacina (*left*) and Fran Nelson express their gratitude while still wearing their Bari hospital robes. Sadly, the Americans soon lost touch with Duffy.

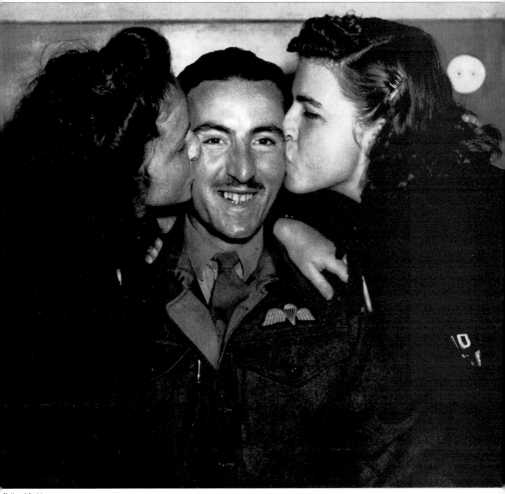

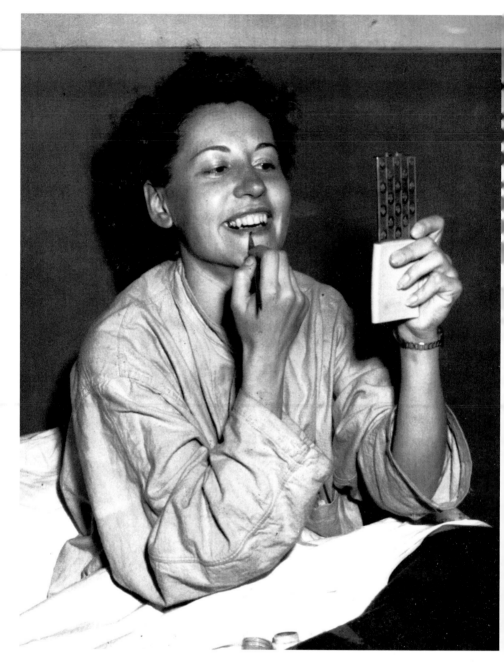

Jean Rutkowski celebrates her rescue by applying lipstick
in her Bari hospital bed. Seven weeks earlier, while scaling
the Albanian Alps amid a blinding blizzard, she fell on the
trail and begged to be left for dead. Her mates pulled her
up and helped her to safety.

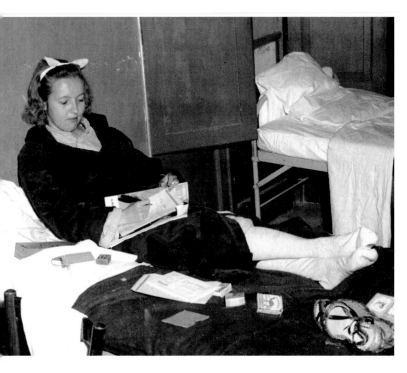

Lois Watson McKenzie puffs on a Camel while scribbling a letter to her parents from the Bari hospital. She waited almost forty years before finally writing a brief memoir of the ordeal.

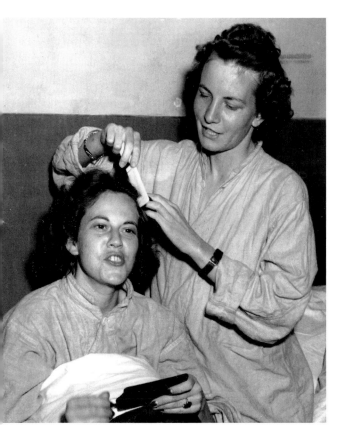

A day or two after their rescue, Agnes Jensen (*right*) combs the hair of Gertrude "Tooie" Dawson in Bari. Tooie and Jens were two of the 807th's senior nurses. Once Albania's Communist regime fell a half century later, Jens finally felt it was okay to publish her memoir, *Albanian Escape*.

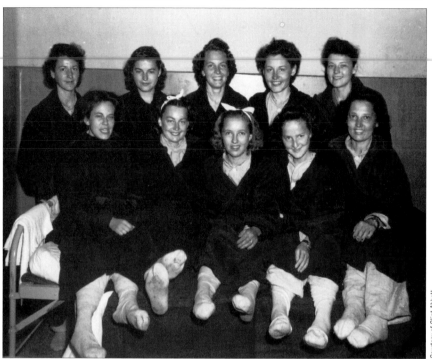

The nurses pose for a photograph at the Bari hospital a day or two after they were rescued, January 1944: (*front row, left to right*): Gertrude "Tooie" Dawson, Elna Schwant, Lois Watson McKenzie, Lillian "Tassy" Tacina, and Ann Kopsco; (*back row, left to right*): Ann Markowitz, Frances Nelson, Agnes "Jens" Jensen, Jean Rutkowski, and Pauleen Kanable.

The noncoms after their rescue (*left to right*): Gilbert Hornsby, Dick Lebo, Charlie Adams, Robert Cranson, Willis Shumway, Paul Allen, Bill Eldridge, Jim Cruise (*lying down*), Raymond Eberg, Harold Hayes, Gordon MacKinnon, Bob Owen, Orville Abbott, Charlie Zeiber, and J. P. Wolf.

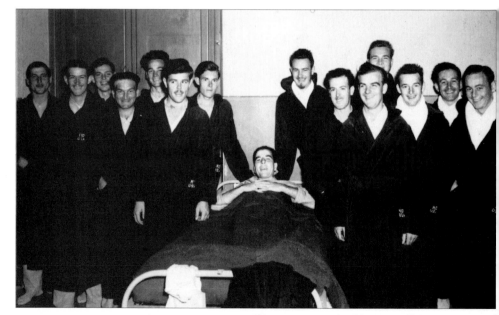

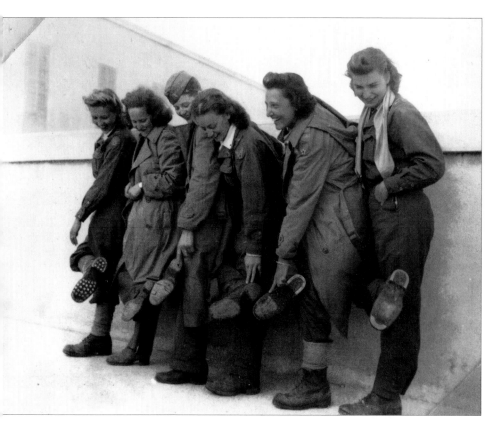

It took five weeks before censors finally allowed welcome-home photos to be distributed to U.S. papers. This is the shot that garnered the biggest play back home— the nurses showing that their boot bottoms had been worn down to the nub: (*left to right*) Lois Watson McKenzie, Lillian Tacina, Paula Kanable, Elna Schwant, Ann Kopsco, and Frances Nelson.

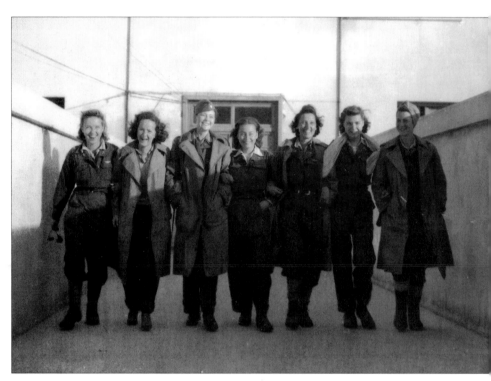

Grinning ear to ear, seven of the nurses locked arms in
Bari: (*left to right*) Lois Watson McKenzie, Lillian Tacina,
Paula Kanable, Elna Schwant, Ann Kopsco, Frances Nelson,
and Ann Markowitz.

Along with Helen Porter, Ann Maness (*left*) and Wilma
Lytle got separated from the rest of the party when the
Germans attacked Berat. They were forced to hide in a
farmhouse for three extra months before Allied intelligence
and friendly Albanians could arranged their rescue. The
unknown guerrilla was one of Tare Shyti's men.

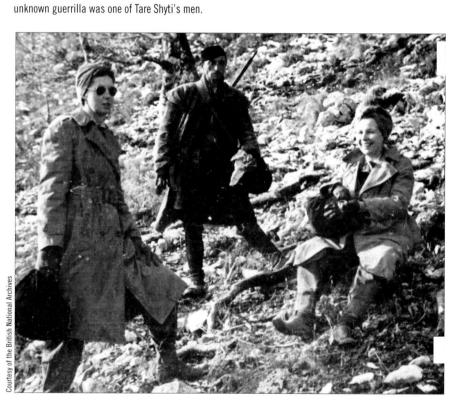

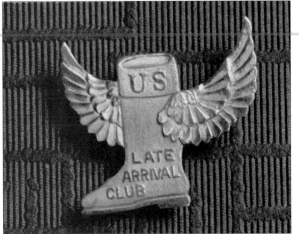

The AAF Late Arrival Club winged boot that Owen and Abbott received in June of 1944 while stationed in Orlando. The boot acknowledged that they had "walked back" after crashing in hostile territory. It was the only U.S. "medal" that Abbott, Owen, or anyone else in the 807th specifically received for their Albanian ordeal.

Together with Elna Schwant Krumm, Orville Abbott's son, Clint (*left*), and Agnes Jensen Mangerich did a presentation and book signing in Newaygo, Michigan, in August 2001, nineteen years after Orville's death. Jens's book came out in 1999; Clint's a decade later.

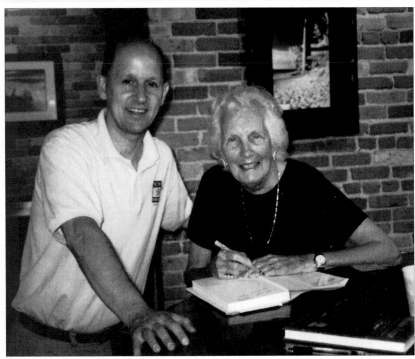

The pilots asked the nurses to guess Duffy's age. Early thirties, maybe? they ventured. No, came the reply, midtwenties. Operating behind enemy lines for seven months while eating and sleeping erratically had taken its toll.

At some point on December 15 or 16, the airmen met with the nurses and medics and told them that they'd hatched a plan to arrange a rescue by air. The deserted airfield that they'd crossed earlier outside Gjirokastër was large enough to handle a C-47 transport. It would be dicey, the airmen said, but right now it looked like their only way out.

Their plan was to have Duffy issue a special operation request via radio to Cairo and Bari. The nurses and medics readily agreed. Everyone was tired of wandering around southern Albania with enemy guns around every bend.

When Duffy resurfaced, the Americans approached him with the idea of being rescued by plane. Abbott remembered the British lieutenant forcefully shaking his head, saying it was too dangerous and unrealistic. But the Americans persisted.

Duffy shot them a dark look, hissing, "We don't know how much of the [radio] stuff we send through is being intercepted. If we tried a scheme like that it jolly well might mean a hot reception for your [Air Force] chaps when they got here. And if it didn't, the Huns would make these people here pay bloody well for letting you get out."

Not wishing to provoke him any further, the Americans let the matter drop—but only temporarily. As each hour passed and their condition became more grave, they were hell-bent on making the air rescue happen. They had no way of knowing, of course, but their plan jibed with what OSS, not to mention their commander in chief, was demanding at that very moment.

Each day, Duffy, Blondie, and sometimes Williamson would disappear for long stretches to communicate with their bosses. Pandee, Steffa, and the other Albanian guides would take point, while the Brits would hustle to catch up after decoding their radio instructions and trying to make sense of the latest intelligence.

By December 17, as they worked their way to a village called Progonat, it was clear that the situation had grown bleaker. On the trail they kept running into refugees, many bruised and bleeding, eyes wild with fear, streaming from one village or another. Steffa and Pandee would translate, but it was always the same story: The Germans were everywhere. Fighting had erupted in all directions. Steffa was especially glum; they kept encountering wounded Partisans, a number of them from a unit that Steffa said he'd helped organize.

By then, Jens could barely hold down food. She was having difficulty keeping up. At one point Abbott and Fran Nelson noticed that Jens was missing from the trail; concerned, they doubled back. Several hundred yards to the rear they found Duffy escorting the American nurse on a mule. She was white as a ghost but attempted a limp smile when asked how she was feeling.

"Garry is a good guy," Nelson said softly to Abbott. "He wouldn't leave anybody behind."

When they reached Progonat, a collection of four or five homes on a once-picturesque plateau that had been savaged by the Germans, the village elders grabbed Pandee for a parley. They were all jabbering at once, shaking their heads.

Pandee walked back to the group to deliver the disheartening news. There was intense fighting along the route they intended to take to the coast.

"A big push," Duffy said resignedly. "They're kicking bloody hell out of the Albanians. There are dead everywhere. Not a mouse could get through those Jerry lines now."

"The Huns had us stopped," Abbott wrote later. "We were washed up. We could climb mountains on our hands and knees, we'd done it; we could live on corn bread and sour milk, we'd done that; we would sleep with the lice and fleas chewing us, march in the rain, and go barefoot if we had to. All these things we could do, while there was ahead of us the hope of the blue sea, the hope of getting back to our lines, the hope of home! Now that hope was gone."

For the first time they all began contemplating the idea of taking their chances with a surrender.

By December 18, OSS Captain Lloyd Smith and his guides had set out for the small southwestern town of Kuç, since Smith had been informed that Duffy and the American group would be there by the twenty-first. But the fighting in the villages along the trail was so fierce that Smith had to turn back and recalculate his route. On the nineteenth, having spent the previous night in a cave along the coast, Smith managed to commandeer an automobile from a guerrilla leader in Vuno. The man baldly predicted that the Partisans were too strong to be uprooted by the Germans in the Kuç region.

Smith's Albanian acquaintance clearly wasn't seeing what Duffy and Blondie were seeing. Duffy and his wireless operator probed Kuç's eastern side on the nineteenth by themselves. The situation was so harrowing that the LNC-SOE outpost in Kuç had been moved east to Golem. Duffy again was forced to recalibrate their path. The Germans were not only on both sides of Kuç, but seemed to be on all sides of everywhere.

Sans Duffy, Blondie, and Williamson on the morning of December 20, the group had been instructed to follow Steffa and the other guides on a convoluted path toward Kuç. It was a gloomy rerun: Every trail was choked with panicked refugees.

The Americans marched, Abbott wrote, "in morose silence, inwardly cursing Adolf Hitler and all Nazis with every step." An hour or so in, they spotted Duffy's woolen beret bobbing above the crowd, heading toward them.

There was too much fighting ahead, Duffy brusquely informed them; they had no choice but to backtrack. Duffy immediately pivoted them 180 degrees and took the point.

Thrasher and Baggs, figuring they had nothing to lose, urged Duffy that day to tell the big bosses to send a plane for them. Duffy, who'd been up all night again, kept walking, but the group could sense his fury.

Jens was close enough to recollect the exchange. "We can't do that," Duffy spat out.

"Why not?" Thrasher countered. "We'll make up a message for you to send out tonight, if you want."

"No, I don't want, and if you send any such message, you will direct it to your own air force headquarters, or whoever may be in command," Duffy replied.

"Well, okay," Baggs responded. "We can address it to Commander of the Twelfth Air Force."

Duffy asked whether they had any idea who that was. "General Spaatz," came the reply.

"I don't mind asking him for a lift on one of his C-47s under these circumstances," Thrasher said.

"I have my orders," Duffy reiterated, "and they are to get you people to the coast safely."

"We'll take responsibility for this," Thrasher said.

"You're damn right you will," Duffy snapped. He then motioned for the pilots, Steffa, and Pandee to stick with him and told the rest of the group to follow the other guides toward Kolonja.

In his report that night, Duffy described the frustration of being only a two-day march from the sea—but not being able to proceed. "The German drive was an avalanche," his report concluded.

Lloyd Smith, meanwhile, was facing his own daunting challenge from Kuç's western side. He got within a few miles of town before being informed that the Germans had captured it earlier that day. Again, he had to adjust his route and strategy.

To further dampen spirits, an ice storm hit that afternoon. It was almost dark by the time the party reached Kolonja, drenched and shivering. It took the guides fifteen minutes of back-and-forth to negotiate a place for them to stay the night. No food was offered. Except for a swallow or two from their canteens, they'd had nothing all day. The blankets they were handed that night felt like oily sandpaper.

They were in the middle of nowhere without their male officers or their protectors, virtually encircled by a revenge-crazed enemy that might well be expressly looking for *them.* The sergeants were able to communicate the danger to the guides, who agreed to maintain sentries around the village all night. If the guards spotted Ballists or Germans moving in, they would fire a shot of warning.

Twice during the night, single shots rang out, causing the Americans to bolt off the cold floor. Both times it was a false alarm: Trigger-happy guards had fired without provocation.

At dawn they were greeted by the specter of an elderly Albanian woman desperate to have them leave her home and village. *"Germani! Germani!"* she kept repeating, while making a slashing motion across her throat.

They tried to explain that they couldn't leave until the rest of the party caught up. Between the lack of food and their guilt over subjecting their hosts to danger, everyone was miserable.

Steffa and the pilots finally arrived around one thirty that afternoon. The group immediately pounced on them about sending them ahead without an English-speaking interpreter. They calmed down when the pilots told them that Duffy had finally allowed them to send a radio message requesting an air rescue. It wasn't a sure thing that the request had gotten through to the right authorities; even if it had, the weather was so bad it wouldn't have made much of a difference.

The weather was still dreadful when Duffy and Blondie joined them after dark. Under the conditions, it was impossible for them to leave Kolonja. Duffy no doubt provided their hostess with some gold for her troubles, but she remained petrified that the Germans were so close.

Still unfed, the group left Kolonja at dawn in a sleet storm. Within minutes, they were chilled to the bone. But they had to hike all day long on Duffy's new route, ending at sunset at a village called Karla.

There, amid the pandemonium of hundreds of other refugees, they saw a familiar mustachioed figure in a cape: It was Hasan Jina. He thumped the men on the back and bussed the women on both cheeks.

He was alarmed to learn that there still had been no word about the three nurses left behind in Berat.

"Too bad to Ann [Maness]," Jens recalled Hasan saying. "I like her very much! Germans are very bad. Maybe I soon teach them a lesson for Ann."

When Jens and the others inquired what Hasan had meant by his bluster, he volunteered that the Germans had a habit of driving their officers around in open staff cars. A well-aimed grenade or stick of dynamite could prove lethal.

What would happen if the Germans caught him? the Americans inquired.

"I throw stick of dynamite and disappear like the wind. I not get caught." He grinned.

The next morning some of the medics happened to be out in the village when Hasan and his band of guerrillas were departing at 0700. They bade him another farewell.

"He lived with danger day and night, accepting the one rule of, 'kill or be killed,' as a matter of course," Abbott wrote. Abbott hoped that one day he would get a chance to repay the debt the group owed Hasan.

Jens, Jean Rutkowski, and Tooie Dawson went looking for Hasan that morning and were upset to learn that he'd already departed.

Duffy had reset their course for Doksat, a village nestled about a mile below Gjirokastër and a short distance from the old Italian airstrip. They were backtracking, in part because there seemed to be fewer Germans in the area and in part because the LNC sympathizers there were better equipped than most Albanians; Duffy was told by Steffa and the guides that food should be plentiful in Doksat. The British lieutenant didn't volunteer it, but they were hunkered down near Gjirokastër to be close to the airfield if a rescue were to be attempted.

Moreover, the group, and not incidentally Duffy himself, needed rest. They were not only exhausted, but mentally fatigued. There had been much internecine squabbling, not only over a potential rescue but over trifling matters. At the last minute as they were leaving Krushove, the Brits had bequeathed to two nurses several cartons of cigarettes. Instead of sharing the smokes, the pair was hoarding them for themselves, which caused considerable friction.

Since there was no food around, tobacco was the only way they had of slaking their appetites.

With tempers running hot, the group needed a break from the trail. The fact that it happened to be near the Christmas holiday was an added bonus. They would stay in Doksat at least a couple of days, Duffy announced.

Doksat was a pleasant-looking place, with trim homes and a cobblestone street. At that point, it hadn't yet been hit by the Germans.

They were separated by rank and sex into different homes. Since it was Christmas Eve, they decided to celebrate the holiday together, as best they could.

The nurses were staying in a comfortable three-story house with a wooden tub. McKenzie got to wash her hair for only the second time in seven weeks—the nicest Christmas gift she could possibly have received. The warm water made them all feel better and put them into a slightly more festive mood.

Someone found a red ribbon in a musette bag and made a Christmas decoration by twining it to a small cedar bough.

At the medics' home, their elderly Albanian hostess got upset at the men for being too boisterous—probably because they'd uncorked some *raki*. Jim Cruise, who believed that the way to calm an angry woman was to kiss her, jumped up and gave her a big Christmas hug. When Johnny Wolf tried the same routine, she tugged her skirt and ran screaming out of the room.

The other men asked Abbott to pull out his prayer book and read aloud a couple of appropriate passages. Abbott chose a traditional Anglican appeal. "'Visit, we beseech Thee, O Lord, this place, and drive from it all the snares of the enemy,'" Abbott read. "'May Thy holy angels dwell herein to keep us in peace, and may Thy blessing be on us always. Amen.'"

The men joined the ladies later that evening. "For many of the young sergeants, this was their first Christmas away from home,"

Jens wrote. "They wondered aloud about their younger brothers and sisters and told of the last time they had watched as the kids tore into their presents."

When they started singing carols, they were surprised that Steffa knew more verses than they did. "Mr. Fultz taught them to us in the American-Albanian school and I never forgot them," he said. "I have taught them to my wife and children, too."

Steffa probably did not know that at that very moment Fultz was celebrating a quiet holiday as a Balkans specialist in OSS's Mediterranean headquarters. Code-named "Gates" and nicknamed *Plak* (Albanian for "old man"), Fultz had been feeding FDR and Donovan privileged information about the episode from its outset.

Many of them teared up as they sang the "all is calm, all is bright" line from "Silent Night," despite kidding one another that it would confuse the Albanians into thinking they were German and singing *Stille Nacht*. Even the impassive Duffy got caught up in sentiment. After two weeks of enigmatic behavior on the trail, he finally shared a few details of his background, including the fact that he'd been born in Dublin.

"You're Irish and yet you're fighting for the Brits?" they razzed him.

Duffy got huge laughs by rejoining, "Let's say we finish this war before we go back to the other, eh?"

After fortifying themselves with more *raki*, they decided to sing "The Star-spangled Banner" just before midnight, then at the Brits' insistence, honored the Crown by singing "God Save the King." The Americans knew the tune, of course, but not the words, so most just hummed along.

Some of them planned to go to Orthodox services at five o'clock the next morning, so they had a short night. For a few precious moments, they thought about something other than the dreadful mess in which they found themselves.

CHAPTER 8

THE AIR RESCUE GOES AWRY

They were still cheerful Christmas morning—even the ones who had gotten up before dawn to sit in unforgiving pews. But as the day wore on the enormity of what they were up against hit them all over again.

"The damper went down," Abbott wrote of the medics' Christmas afternoon. "We were ragged, tired, hungry, lousy, unshaven, and dirty."

There wasn't enough tobacco among the noncoms to roll a single cigarette. Not even light-fingered Bill Eldridge's thieving of a yule log could lift them out of their doldrums.

That night, they tried to fight off the gloom by gathering at the male officers' home and sharing a meal that astonishingly included a little fried chicken, rice soup, chopped liver, figs, nuts, and some kind of candied delicacy. Duffy and his deep pockets also had managed to acquire a bottle of vermouth, two bottles of wine, and a jug of *raki*. Their hostesses showed the Americans a Tosk dance that several of the ladies attempted, some solo, some with male partners.

The Americans were eager to find out whether there had been any wireless updates regarding a potential rescue or a break in the fighting. But no one dared to unloose Duffy's temper.

Duffy admitted that night that it had taken him a while to get used to being around so many women. None of his siblings were girls; he found the entire gender a bit baffling.

Jens responded that he'd certainly gotten a crash course in the ways of women, which induced chuckles all around.

"I must admit that when I was first given the assignment to evacuate a group that included ten nurses, I almost turned tail and ran," Jens heard Duffy saying. "However, when I met you and learned that you had already been through quite a bit since you crash-landed and were still in good spirits, I felt sure—God willing—that I could get you to the coast.

"You know, you girls really have a lot of guts."

That intestinal fortitude would be severely tested in the days to come. Duffy didn't share it Christmas night, but he knew operational planning for an air rescue was well under way. He still didn't like it, but the matter—at least for the moment—was out of his hands.

"We Brits underestimated the power of the president [Roosevelt]," B8 intelligence chief Naar wrote sixty-nine years later. "Leaving no stone unturned, and without consulting us, FDR came up with a completely different plan of action: a *force majeure*, a show of force, American-style. It was, one of our OSS associates jokingly quipped, 'time to send in the Marines.'"

FDR and the American military didn't summon the Marines. But they sent in practically everyone else—subtlety, subterfuge, and the opinions of the Allied intelligence professionals in the field be damned.

Naar and his B8 colleagues first got wind of the Americans' grand scheme some ten days after Naar got chewed out by FDR and immediately after Thrasher and Baggs had issued their radio plea to General Carl Spaatz. By then the Balkan SOE headquarters had moved from Cairo to Bari, just across the Adriatic from the clandestine operations it was running in Albania, Yugoslavia, and elsewhere.

The dramatic plan to swoop a U.S. plane into Albania to pick up the stranded Americans was presented to Leake, Naar, and the Brits essentially as a fait accompli. Naar, relying on Duffy's terse reports, warned OSS and the Allied air forces that heavily armed Germans were now ensconced throughout southern Albania and were in control of the few airfields there. The enemy was also no doubt aware that the American refugees were in their midst. With Nazi artillery and armor uncomfortably close, it would be too hazardous to attempt an air rescue, Leake, Naar, and Duffy argued. The old Italian runway near Gjirokastër was tucked in a valley; it wouldn't take much for the enemy to train guns on it.

Moreover, Naar reminded his American counterparts, Bari and its airfield, the place where the operation would originate, were rife with Nazi spies. Too many Allied servicepeople had already been clued in to the raid's lengthy logistical preparations; there was a strong likelihood that the Germans in Albania would be tipped off. Even if the enemy didn't have advance knowledge, the air rescue plan was fraught with danger. The percentage move, the Brits maintained, was to stick to *their* plan of marching the party to the Adriatic coast.

It all fell on deaf ears. None of the American higher-ups would listen. Clearly, the Yanks were reacting to explicit orders from the top—in this case, the very top. An impatient FDR was getting regular updates from Donovan and Fultz. He wanted the "flower of American womanhood" rescued—and he didn't want to hear talk about how risky the operation might be.

The greater danger, in FDR's mind, was to sit back and do nothing, knowing that at any instant, the nurses and medics could be snatched by the enemy. From the president's point of view, the SOE had been leading the Americans through the mountains of Albania for the better part of a month—with little to show for it. The group was no closer to freedom on Christmas Day than it had been in early December. The U.S. top brass thought it was time to try something different other than hiking the group up and down the Albanian Alps.

The American high command's decision making was also driven by its frustrations over OSS's inability to reach the stranded Americans. On the day after Christmas, Lloyd Smith, still bottled up west of Kuç, received orders to turn around: There were too many Germans between him and Doksat. Smith's two and a half weeks of trying to circumvent the German offensive and get to the evaders had proven fruitless.

FDR and his intelligence people wanted the 807th out of Albania, come hell or high water. And they didn't care how many planes it would take out of service from the Allied air forces.

On the afternoon of December 26, as Lloyd Smith headed back across the Adriatic, the group spent another quiet day in Doksat praying for a break in the soupy weather. None came. Nor was there further word about a possible rescue. Their depression kicked in all over again.

The next morning, as the nurses looked out their windows, it was clear the village was buzzing—but the women didn't know

why. At noontime, they found out when an agitated Duffy barged
in and asked to be taken to the house's top floor, where he could
look at Gjirokastër through his field glasses.

He'd never be able to see anything, they told Duffy as he took
the steps two at a time. But when they reached the top floor and
craned their necks out the transom, they realized that there had
indeed been a slight break in the clouds.

The rumors running rampant through the village were correct,
Duffy told them: The Germans had moved into Gjirokastër in a
big way. Through his binoculars he could see motorcycles, jeeps,
half-tracks, trucks pulling antiaircraft and antitank guns, and even
tanks moving into the village. It was all a retaliation, Duffy casually noted, for a staff car full of German officers who'd been killed
a day or two earlier.

Duffy's revelation jarred Jens and the nurses: It was Hasan's
prophecy come to life. Had Hasan made good on his threat to blow
up enemy officers to avenge his friend, the missing Ann Maness?
The Americans never found out for certain. But the German move
into Gjirokastër, they all understood, could fatally jeopardize their
chances of getting away. The airfield they wanted to use for the
rescue was now within a few minutes' drive of heavy Nazi firepower.

Duffy still didn't breathe a word, but the air rescue operation
was now scheduled to go the instant the weather cleared. He
immediately began sending urgent messages to Naar about the
strength and proximity of the enemy force. Duffy suspected that
his protests would be ignored; nevertheless, he was trying to avert
what he feared would be a bloodbath.

Three of the American sergeants had managed to acquire binoculars; all day long on the twenty-seventh they took turns from
the perch in the nurses' house to watch enemy vehicles climb the
perilous road toward Gjirokastër's ancient Ottoman fortress, fearing that at any minute the Germans would send motorcycles and

an assassination squad into Doksat. By the end of the day, beyond learning that the German unit had been based in Delvinë, a few miles closer to the Greek border, Duffy didn't know any more about enemy intentions in Gjirokastër than he'd known at noon.

Still, it didn't look good; the Germans clearly intended to stay for the foreseeable future. Almost as troubling, the weather was causing Blondie and Williamson's wireless to act up again. At eight o'clock that night the Brits tried to reach Cairo or Bari, with no luck. Duffy worried that the Germans were jamming their circuits.

When told that their radio was temperamental, Elna Schwant lamented that it was radio trouble and lousy weather that had gotten them into their quandary in the first place.

The nurses were trying to sip bony goat soup at lunchtime on December 28 when Thrasher and Baggs came calling.

Since the weather was breaking, it was official, they said. Duffy had just gotten word that a C-47, maybe two, probably escorted by fighter planes, would be attempting to rescue them the following day.

The nurses were floored.

"Do you mean it? You wouldn't kid us now, would you?" one of them allowed, according to Jens.

It was very real, they were assured. Duffy was confirming details with SOE Bari, reiterating his concerns about the amount of German armor next door. But orders were orders. The British lieutenant wanted everyone in the party to steel themselves. To have any chance of success, the rescue demanded complete cooperation and discipline, he emphasized.

The medics were also euphoric, but there was great concern that Duffy was so opposed to the rescue that, even now, he would try to scrub it.

Saturday morning, December 29, dawned clear and mild— the best weather southern Albania had seen in more than a week.

Naar and the Brits, who had been begging the USAAF for months to lend them planes to drop arms and supplies to the Partisans, were dumbstruck at the firepower the Americans had assembled at the Bari airfield. It was, Naar remembers, "a veritable armada": thirty-six P-38 Lockheed Lightning fighter planes, two C-47 Dakota transports, and one Wellington bomber on loan from the British Balkan Air Force. The Wellington was supposed to land first, swinging its nose, rear, and waist-side machine guns to return hostile fire.

"To us Brits," Naar wrote, "the whole affair seemed more like a Hollywood movie than a seriously workable plan of action." SOE clung to a slim hope that the scheme was so far-fetched it might catch the Germans napping.

Naar and his team drove out to the Bari airfield early on the morning of the twenty-ninth to watch the armada get mobilized. The Brits couldn't help but enjoy a moment of schadenfreude when, at the last minute, the raid's U.S. commander tripped on his pretentiously long aviator's scarf, badly spraining his ankle as he attempted to climb into the cockpit of his P-38. Only one pilot was available in Bari to replace the commander, a laconic New Zealander. Between the Kiwi fighter jock and the critical Wellington bomber crew, the Royal Air Force was suddenly well represented on the raid.

An outsider unfamiliar with the mission's nuances, therefore, was now at least partly responsible for leading the raiders over the target. But the armada bought a couple of early breaks that morning: The weather was passable, no ack-ack came their way, and no bevy of German fighters scrambled to challenge them en route. It was a flight of only about 140 miles; in less than an hour they managed to find the southeastern corner of Albania and with it, the old airstrip outside Gjirokastër.

Duffy remained wary but still had a job to do. The weather continued to cooperate; there was a little ground haze but it would soon dissipate, thanks to an unseasonably warm sun.

At daybreak, he gathered the group together. With Thrasher and Baggs chiming in, he walked them through the blow-by-blow of the rescue operation. In late morning, they would move within a few hundred yards of the airfield but stay concealed in the woods. The planes were expected sometime between noon and one o'clock. They would have to scramble quickly, because the noise was sure to alert the enemy. Five men—it turned out to be Abbott, Hayes, Lebo, Shumway, and Wolf—would run out onto the field when the planes arrived and signal the pilots by waving parachute panels. To guarantee that no one would be weighted down, they would leave all their equipment with the Partisans.

Moreover, to distract potential enemy shooters as the planes touched down, Duffy wanted two separate groups running toward the transports from different directions. The transports would be on the ground for only a few seconds, he stressed. It would be up to each of them to gauge where the planes would be coming to a stop—and adjust their running accordingly. The side cargo doors would be open; airmen inside would reach out and pull the runners aboard. Once everyone had been accounted for, the planes would quickly turn around and take off.

The men in each group, Thrasher gratuitously added, would be responsible for ensuring that the women got to the planes safely.

"That means," Abbott quoted Thrasher as opining with a sardonic grin, "that you get them there alive and no broken bones!" Tooie Dawson spoke for all the nurses when she assured the male officers that the women could more than take care of themselves.

But even she softened when Thrasher said he'd been authorized to tell them that the 807th's "Old Man," Major Red McKnight, would be on one of the transports. They all cheered. Bob

Owen promptly threatened to kiss McKnight, bristly mustache and all.

They all understood the danger, Abbott recalled, but spirits were soaring. A little before 1100, Duffy led them toward the field, positioning them behind a low hill with thick brush cover. Their hiding spot was some three hundred yards removed from the strip, down a severe slope. For more than an hour, they knelt, waiting. Somebody stage-whispered that it was high noon; their hearts began palpitating all over again.

At about 1220, one of the Partisans got Thrasher's attention. The two had a private and clearly unhappy conversation, full of disconsolate gestures. As the Partisan returned to his position, Thrasher signaled for the group to assemble.

Thrasher was so upset he had trouble getting the words out. Finally he explained that the messenger had been sent by Duffy, who was farther up the hill, keeping the Germans in Gjirokastër under surveillance.

The news was not good: It was as if the enemy knew the armada was coming. Several 88mm dual ack-ack/field artillery guns and Panzers had been moved into position almost on top of the airfield.

It was too late to radio the planes and have them turn back, but Duffy was still calling off the rescue. There would be no signaling for the transports to land, Thrasher said; it was too risky.

Some in the party began cursing and wailing, especially when Duffy surfaced a few moments later, toting his machine gun, his eyes black with anger. Bob Owen immediately volunteered that he didn't care about the risk; he was more than willing to take his chances. Other chimed in, too.

"Sorry," Abbott had Garry responding. "It wouldn't make the least difference if every one of us was killed, but it happens that the price in planes and the men who fly them would be too high."

The protests mounted, but Duffy continued to shake his head, insisting it would be a slaughter if he allowed the planes to land.

A few minutes later they heard the buzz of incoming airplanes. Despite their heartache, the Americans started jumping up and down, just as they had forty-seven days earlier when they witnessed the B-25 bombing assault on the Berat-Kuçovë airfield.

"Then we saw them," Abbott wrote later, still moved by what he witnessed that December afternoon. "The bright sun flashing on their wings, wings that carried the beloved markings. . . . Two C-47 transports with the great stars blazing white on their sleek sides. A big Wellington bomber that zoomed low over the village like a bully, spoiling for a fight, daring the Jerries to open up." The enemy guns stayed silent.

Jens remembered three P-38 fighter-bombers screeching so low across the field that it felt like she could touch them. As they pulled up, one flew straight on, and the other two fanned out in opposite directions—one over Gjirokastër and the other right over [the enemy's] heads. Three more followed in a beautifully precise formation as the first three fell in at the rear for another pass."

The two C-47s had already gone wheels-down and were clearly looking for the ground signal to land. Within seconds, they pulled up and joined the P-38s in a majestic circle of the field. The Americans were sure that the pilots could see them jumping and waving.

The nurses and medics marveled at the pilots' precision. "You'd have thought they were playing tag around the old home pasture," Charlie Adams said to Abbott. "They seemed to know every foot of the place. [The pilots] must have been briefed for hours."

Duffy's charges were bellowing like banshees, clawing at him, pleading with him to let them execute the landing signal. His jaw set, he kept cursing and shaking his head.

"How our military discipline held us at that point, I don't know," admitted Abbott. The planes kept circling as the Americans on the ground groveled.

Finally, Duffy relented.

"His nod was all we needed," Abbott remembered. "Behind us

as we took off, we heard him yell, 'Cover!' as he shoved his gun at one of his sergeants. Then [Duffy] was running with us. We tore our parachute scarves from our necks as we went. It was like running a 440 at the state meet. . . . It was murder. Our bodies were dying, numb with the swift ebb of our strength; we had only a savage will somewhere inside that kept us going."

Savage will or no, they didn't make it. By the time the five signalers and Duffy got up to the field, the planes were winging northwest, back toward Bari.

"They were gone," Abbott wrote. "We had lost the race. We lay flat on the ground, fighting for our breath, our hearts bursting, sobbing our despair, feeling like we were going to die, and wanting to." Many of the nurses, including McKenzie, collapsed as they wept.

Later they learned that the armada's trip to Albania was not completely in vain. As the gaggle headed toward the Strait of Otranto, the pilots spotted a convoy of enemy trucks. The P-38s tore the German caravan to shreds.

But the group knew nothing of this as they contemplated their fate. At that instant they all hated Duffy for holding them up so long that it queered the mission. Utterly dejected, they picked themselves off the ground. They had no choice but to hurry back to Doksat—the Germans could be on their tail.

Despite it all, it didn't take long for them to realize that Duffy had been right. Had the bomber and the transports landed, the enemy guns almost certainly would have opened fire, Baggs and Thrasher agreed. There was no element of surprise; everyone could have been mowed down. The German gunners probably didn't fire because they wanted the big planes to touch down before exposing their positions.

As they trudged toward the village, tears continued to well in Lois's and Jens's eyes. It humbled them that the Allied command would go to such great risk for twenty-seven anonymous soldiers.

To Jens, Duffy, too, seemed on the verge of sobbing.

The lieutenant's after-action report captured the pathos and frustration.

> The nurses had unquestionably suffered a very hard time—this was indeed too much. The planes flew around for over 15 minutes, but I would not bring them in; never in my whole life have I been faced with such a decision. If I had brought them in, here was the picture: three heavy planes on the air field and the Germans not 500 yards away with tanks and guns! Did the Germans fire! At the planes, no! Would they have fired at stationary planes, who knows? I was certainly not going to have three planes jeopardized. Maybe the first plane might have made it, who knows! But I am sure that the other two would not, and my job was to escort and deliver twenty-seven bodies, not a third of the party.

His closing lines betrayed his remorse. "I was in charge of the party and entirely responsible. You can be well assured as recent events have shown. One has a full-time job looking after oneself in Albania without having attachments, female or otherwise." The stoical Duffy had, despite himself, become emotionally involved in his mission.

He and his "attachments, female or otherwise," now had to summon the courage—one more time—to figure out how they were going to avert the Nazi forces that stood between them and freedom.

"Walking back on that trail," Abbott wrote, "I think we began to find the determination to do it. We were going to keep going as long as we could put one foot ahead of the other foot."

The FDR/OSS great gamble had not paid off. In fact, it may

well have backfired, by giving the enemy a road map to the Americans' position.

As discouraged as they were, the Americans were comforted by one thought: "Duffy knew more about fighting Nazis than any ten of us," Abbott wrote.

CHAPTER 9

CRAWLING AROUND THE ENEMY

*Their hosts in Doksat were stunned when the Ameri-*cans abruptly reappeared. With the Germans so close, the people had been relieved that morning when the Americans departed. The villagers, not unreasonably, had assumed the visitors were gone for good. Then there was all the tumult with the Allied warplanes, which had sent bewildered residents scurrying for cover. And now the Americans and their British compadres were back, their binoculars trained on every enemy move up the hill in Gjirokastër.

Duffy and the pilots convened a council to review options. For the time being they would continue to plan for a possible rescue by air, Duffy said. Yet one reality intruded above all others: The Germans on the hilltop almost certainly knew that the lost Americans were in the immediate vicinity. The group had no choice but to vacate as quickly as they could. In the meantime, they would have to maintain constant surveillance so that the enemy couldn't sneak up on them or send hit squads to Doksat or Kesovrat, the adjoining village where some of the men had spent the previous night.

Bill Eldridge, Raymond Eberg, and an Albanian interpreter drew the first watch on December 30, sneaking along the path to Gjirokastër and concealing themselves in the woods. All day long, they watched German motorcycle couriers and jeeps full of soldiers move in and out of the village.

The following day, December 31, Abbott and his fast friend Gilbert Hornsby drew the watch. They sleuthed to a spot that afforded a bird's-eye view of where they'd hidden two days before. A steady stream of enemy motorized equipment moved to and from town.

They had been hiding in the trees for about two hours, careful not to let the sun reflect off their field glasses, when Hornsby nudged Abbott. The Kentuckian was bird-dogging a German jeep that had left the main road, crossed a small bridge, and was now heading across the field toward their position. Abbott snagged the binoculars and brought the jeep into focus.

"There was the German car, moving directly towards us, three Nazis in their field grey uniforms and bucket helmets, the slim black snouts of rifles or Tommy guns sticking up beyond the shoulders of the two men who were riding," Abbott wrote. "They were still several hundred yards from us and I tossed the glasses across the little space to the Albanian, motioning for him to look the car over. Hornsby and I, in the meantime, kept our eyes glued on it.

"'I don't think they've spotted us,' I whispered. The air was cold and crisp, and the words seemed to echo out over the valley like a shout.

"'They'll blow us to hell,' was Hornsby's encouraging reply."

The jeep ground to a halt thirty or forty yards away.

The three men lay motionless, afraid to take a deep breath for fear that the Germans would be able to hear it.

Two of the enemy soldiers eventually left the jeep to intercept Albanians heading in both directions on the path. Each villager was harshly questioned, then allowed to proceed. The Germans spent twenty minutes hassling locals before jumping back into the jeep and retracing their steps to Gjirokastër.

Abbott and Hornsby instructed their guide to track down the villagers, find out why the Germans had interrogated them and what the enemy soldiers were asking. The two Americans, meanwhile, stayed put to maintain the watch.

At one point a truck full of Germans stopped at a farmhouse down the road. Hornsby and Abbott watched through their binoculars as several soldiers got out and ransacked the place; each eventually grabbed a sheep and they tossed the animals into the back of the truck.

The Albanian guide returned. The villagers reported that the Germans wanted to know whether any roads led to Doksat or Kesovrat, and whether people had seen suspicious activity in either place. Breaking out into a "cold sweat," Hornsby and Abbott sent the messenger to warn Duffy and the others.

"At any moment we expected to see a German patrol setting out from Gjirokastër and heading our way," Abbott wrote.

At three o'clock a Partisan fighter crawled to their position, telling them that Duffy wanted them to report back to Doksat right away: The group was pulling out.

Duffy had decided it was too dicey for them to stay close to Gjirokastër. The villagers were understandably nervous about running out of food and terrified at the prospect of the Germans

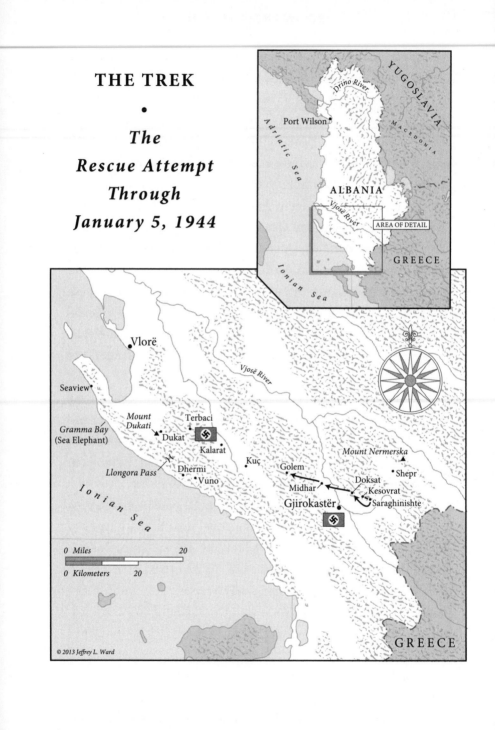

THE TREK

•

The
Rescue Attempt
Through
January 5, 1944

YUGOSLAVIA

Drino River

Port Wilson

Adriatic Sea

MACEDONIA

ALBANIA

Vjosë River

AREA OF DETAIL

GREECE

Ionian Sea

•Vlorë

Vjosë River

Seaview•

Mount
Dukati

Terbaci

Gramma Bay
(Sea Elephant)

•Dukat

Kalarat

Mount Nermerska

Kuç

Golem

•Shepr

Llongora Pass

Dhermi•
•Vuno

Doksat

Midhar

Kesovrat

Ionian Sea

Gjirokastër•

Saraghinishte

0 Miles   20

0 Kilometers   20

© 2013 Jeffrey L. Ward

GREECE

finding out that they'd been harboring Allied fugitives. It was a miracle that somebody hadn't already ratted them out.

By the time Duffy gathered everyone, including a fourteen-year-old Albanian guide, it was almost dark. He explained that it was too dangerous for them to take the regular path to the SOE outpost in Saraghinishte. They'd have to take a cross-country route.

It was rugged going in the gloom. They constantly banged into trees and rocks, scraped shins and knees, and bruised their faces while negotiating thick briar patches.

"From time to time," Abbott recalled, "we crawled on our hands and knees along ledges hardly wide enough for the passage of our bodies, the rough shoulder of the mountain crowding us from one side and a sheer drop of unknown depth on the other. It was a nightmare of effort that seemed never to end and when, suddenly, we found ourselves at our destination, we were amazed to learn that it was still early in the evening."

Saraghinishte was a cluster of a half dozen homes, nicely appointed by Albanian standards. When Jens, Lois, Markie, and the others arrived at their designated house for the evening, they watched with curiosity as their host family buried a large trunk in their side yard. Jens and company quickly deduced that the trunk contained family heirlooms and valuables. The people of Saraghinishte did not want to have happen to them what had happened to the denizens of Berat and dozens of other Albanian villages—to be plundered by the Germans. The digging had been done so discreetly, its top covered by grass and rocks, that the next morning the women could hardly tell that the ground had been excavated.

No doubt enriched by a few of Duffy's sovereigns, their host families broke all records for hospitality, Abbott remembered.

Jens and her group of nurses were served a pot of fatty goat stew; one whiff caused Jens to feel nauseated all over again. Even the sound of the others' spoons hitting the side of the pot made what was left of her stomach flip-flop.

They almost forgot it was New Year's Eve. But when somebody remembered, it triggered a flood of memories. Exactly one year earlier, Jens had been on call at the Fort Benning hospital, which meant, unlike her nursing friends, she didn't have to worry about showing up at a gala party in uniform. This year, she told her pals, she'd be thrilled to wear any uniform to a party, as long as it was clean.

McKenzie admitted she'd never really cared for her mother's holiday eggnog and fruitcake—but she'd give anything to go to the Watsons' New Year's Day open house in Oak Lawn.

The holiday talk made Elna Schwant grow quiet. Just before they had boarded the *Santa Elena* four months earlier, Elna had gotten a letter from her father with the sad news that her brother, a Navy pilot in the Pacific theater, had been declared missing in action. By now, no doubt, her folks had gotten word that she was missing, too. There were two other Schwant children in the service: a younger daughter who was a WAC and a younger son, also in the Army. Both were on active duty somewhere, so it would be a difficult holiday for the Schwant family of Winner, South Dakota.

The men, meanwhile, fantasized about what New Year's Eve at home would be like, with "lights, laughter, girls, food, drink, dancing, the funny hats, the paper horns, streamers of bright colored tissue floating over the celebrating crowd, confetti showering everyone as the hour of the New Year struck," Abbott wrote.

But they weren't back in the States or even in the friendly confines of Catania. They were in God-knew-where Albania, having just crawled over a mountain to avoid Nazi patrols and ruthless Barleys.

Captain Lloyd Smith spent New Year's in a shepherd's cave not far from the small German U-boat base at Grava Bay. Smith had now been trying to reach the stranded Americans for some five weeks.

Yet he was still many miles removed. He was using guides to bribe their fellow Ballis to look the other way and allow safe passage. But he knew neither the country nor the nefarious— and thoroughly corrupt—ways of BK mercenaries. Even after the Germans retreated, he was counting his progress in yards, not miles.

On New Year's night in Saraghinishte the male officers hosted a get-together; given the bleak circumstances, spirits were buoyant as they toasted getting the hell out of Albania.

An air rescue was almost definitely off, Duffy told the group. They were still too close to the German encampment at Gjirokastër; another air armada would risk bringing the hordes upon them. This time they might not get away so easily.

Their path to the coast was opening up, Duffy's sources in the LNC and SOE were now saying. They would stay in Saraghinishte for at least another day or two. Major Tilman in Shepr had just received fresh supplies via parachute—including new boots and clean clothes for at least some of them. Tilman was arranging for the stuff to be delivered.

Duffy also relayed word that OSS captain Smith was trying to split the difference between their location and the shoreline. The Brit may not have known that Smith at that moment was in Dhermi, well west of Kuç, where he'd used the cache of money he'd been given to hire six guides. Smith directed them to head inland in groups of two, pursuing three different paths. If any of the pairs should encounter the wayward Americans, they were under orders to have one man stay with the party while the other was to report back to Smith. One pair hiked toward Terbaci; another went in the direction of Vranishti and Kalarat; and the other duo trudged toward Kuç and Golem—the very destinations that Smith had for weeks been trying in vain to reach.

Smith's subordinates all shoved off on January 2, which happened to be the moment the Americans enjoyed their day off in Saraghinishte. Several of the medics, Abbott included, were delighted when Tilman's delivery arrived and their new shirts ended up more or less fitting. Even better, the noncoms' host family produced a wooden tub and something akin to soap. For the first time in many days, the men had a decent scrub.

"With our new clothes over our clean bodies and the inner man well satisfied for the first time in weeks, we felt like a million bucks," Abbott recounted.

They spent more time meeting with Duffy to review the drill for heading west. To plow a path forward and arrange for accommodations, Duffy late on the second sent Steffa, Thrasher, and some Albanian guides out ahead. Duffy hoped the pathfinders would save time and aggravation by surveying the trail for signs of the enemy and bartering for places to stay in friendly villages. The less the group could meander—the straighter their shot to the coast—the better. At that point, as the crow flies, they were not far from the Adriatic. But they'd have to surmount one mountain after another and, inevitably, zig and zag to avoid the Germans.

Lois McKenzie questioned Duffy about the location of the German forces and how they would circumvent them. "Couldn't we skirt the areas they're in?" McKenzie asked, maybe a bit too naively.

Annoyed, Duffy responded, "Perhaps, when we find out *where* those are!" That was why he was sending Steffa and Thrasher out ahead, he explained. Even the outspoken McKenzie got the idea that the lieutenant was in no mood for further colloquy.

As Duffy left the conclave he motioned for Jens to follow him outside. Perhaps with McKenzie's exchange top of mind, he asked about the Americans' physical and mental health and their capacity to handle another wearying march. Jens reported that their bouts of dysentery seemed to be receding, but she was worried about Elna Schwant's jaundice, Jim Cruise's cough, and Willis Shumway's knee.

There was clearly something else on Duffy's mind. He fumbled around for the right words, stammering something about certain women being "difficult" because that thing that was supposed to happen once a month maybe wasn't. Duffy was trying to say that many of the women were suffering the effects of amenorrhea; their menstrual cycles had apparently stopped within weeks of the crash.

"Oh, that!" Jens remembered responding. Yes, it was true, she confirmed: Most of the women were no longer menstruating, and few had packed tampons in Catania. But now it was Jens's turn to narrow her eyes.

"Garry," she recalled snapping, "that's an excuse used by some women for their crossness, crying, or just about anything they don't want to take responsibility for—since time immemorial. All I can say is, I've never heard of anyone dying from it, and like everything else that's wrong with us right now, there's not a darn thing we can do about it. Frankly, I consider it one of the few blessings on this jaunt!"

Duffy looked so relieved that for a second Jens thought he was going to give her a kiss. But he backed away, muttering something about wanting to get the group back on the trail as quickly as possible.

"Oh, I do hope so," Jens recalled saying. "If nothing else, there is less quarreling when we're on the move."

In the report he filed on the night of January 2, Duffy acknowledged that the hospitality of the people of Saraghinishte had come with a price: He had doled out copious amounts of sovereigns. His dispatch also expressed hope that by his sending Thrasher and Steffa ahead, they might encounter OSS captain Smith in the vicinity of Kuç or Kalarat, some dozen miles northwest.

The next evening, Duffy announced that they would hit the trail at 0800 on January 4. He told them he was working hard to get mules to lighten the load.

Most of the Americans did not realize the lengths to which Duffy had gone to grease the villagers. As they gathered at 0745, their hosts, on the verge of tears, hugged them and wished them well.

"If we had saved the town from the devil himself they couldn't have made more over us," Abbott recalled. Two days of rest and decent nourishment had worked wonders. They were hell-bent to get out of the mountains.

With an unexpectedly warm sun at their backs, they pushed northwest, hiking as fast as they ever had. Duffy had already warned that German patrols would be combing the two main roads up ahead; at times, he stressed, the group would be relegated to cross-country paths that only the native guides knew about.

The mules helped. During a break that morning, Elna Schwant mischievously pulled some corn bread out of her bosom, borrowed a knife, and began dividing it into small squares. The knife broke through the crust and left Elna with a nasty gash on her thigh. Markie and Harold Hayes grabbed the first-aid kit and patched her up. Elna wanted to walk but Duffy insisted that she ride.

They were going so hard that they arrived four hours ahead of schedule in the village where Steffa and Thrasher had wired accommodations. All agreed that they should continue pushing on. But Duffy, relaying reports from his scouts, said that enemy soldiers were in the vicinity; it was too dangerous to be out in daylight. So they waited a couple of hours, wolfed down a meal of goat soup and corn bread, then got back on the trail close to sundown.

Soon it was spitting frigid rain. In ghostly darkness, they groped their way down a slippery trail. Duffy kept hissing at them to stay quiet and forbade smoking or the use of matches or flashlights. German patrols were everywhere.

After two hours, soaked to the bone, they came upon a big river, probably the Devoll, which they had crossed downstream, heading the other direction, weeks earlier. The scouts had arranged for a barge owner to ferry the group across the stream, since at that juncture it was too wide and deep to ford.

It was so unearthly quiet that a whisper sounded like a shout. Abbott recalled the moon peeking out from behind the clouds. Everyone was crouched at the river's edge, praying the skiff would come and that an enemy patrol wouldn't.

Just then they heard the unmistakable *crack!* of a rifle shot coming from behind them. They flattened themselves on the mucky riverbank, especially when a second *crack!*, then a third, echoed through the woods.

Duffy took a quick head count and realized that Baggs, who was carrying a rifle, was not among them. Baggs all evening had been manning the tail-end position in the column, guarding their backs.

Abbott remembered Duffy whispering that if Baggs had encountered a German patrol, the enemy would not have given the copilot a chance to use his gun.

The group waited with bated breath. Either Baggs or enemy infantry would soon be emerging from the woods.

"At any moment from those murky depths, a blast of fire might come that would cut us down," Abbott remembered. "We didn't relish the idea of plunging off into the unknown woods with an unknown number of armed Nazis on our trails. Garry darted to the edge of the river, his figure a black silhouette against the dull silver of the water."

After what seemed like an eternity, they heard a familiar drawl call out, "If we had some dogs we'd have a coon hunt if there were any coon around here. Damn good night for it."

Baggs soon appeared, rifle slung over his shoulder, grinning a Southern-boy grin.

"What about those shots?" Duffy demanded, not amused by Baggs's good-ol'-boy routine.

Baggs said that he'd fired three rounds as a signal, apparently meaning to intend that he was nearby and that they shouldn't be startled when he came walking out of the woods.

The copilot had been inexcusably careless; unauthorized use of a firearm in such circumstances was a serious breach of conduct, especially for an officer. Duffy stared at Baggs. The group braced for a tirade. But Duffy must have bitten his lip and decided that a riverbank in southern Albania was not the place to dress down someone who, after all, shared his rank. But between Thrasher's joy-hunting of birds amid BK country and Baggs's inexplicable "signal" shots with enemy patrols all around, Duffy must have wondered what kind of military training the USAAF had provided its pilots.

The barge suddenly appeared. Pandee, the lead Albanian guide, gestured for the men to take off their hats, which might make a tempting target as they crossed the river.

It could handle only sixteen people at a time. They went in two groups, with the ten nurses, Baggs, and the Brits going first, followed by the noncoms and the Albanian guides. They all made it across. The slimy river water in the bottom of the barge made their feet even colder.

One of the patrolled roads was dead ahead, so Duffy ordered total silence and demanded that they stay closely bunched. Their luck held.

"The road lay dark and deserted under the blanket of heavy cloud that had now blacked out the moon," Abbott wrote.

They skipped across and found refuge in a gully on the far side. There they caught their breath. Duffy, feeling better, even allowed them to light guarded cigarettes and talk in near-normal tones.

It didn't take them long to reach a village Jens and Duffy recorded as Midhar, a settlement that had been shredded by the Germans. It was so late that there was no sign of life.

Pandee and the other guides began calling out the Tosk equivalent of "Helloooo. . . ." It sounded like a tribal chant out of the Stone Age, Abbott thought. It took a full ten minutes, with Duffy grumbling in between wails, but it worked. Two elders emerged. The nurses, Baggs, and the Brits stayed in Midhar; the enlisted men were escorted to another settlement a full hour's hike away. It was hardly an ideal setup, especially since the men wearing new boots were suffering from blisters.

A guide named Mohamet led the medics down a narrow path to the next village. Mohamet was terrified of being tortured by the BK; he wasn't happy that he would be in charge of negotiating accommodations. He feigned sickness so he wouldn't have to initiate the chant and draw scrutiny on himself.

The Americans were at a loss as to how to get the attention of the villagers. Abbott and company lit a bonfire, another dubious move that would have drawn a stern rebuke from Duffy had he been around. They were so exhausted that no one was thinking clearly.

Eventually, the fire induced some nervous Albanians to leave their homes; fortunately, the smoke wasn't spotted by hostile forces. By now it was only a few hours before dawn. The noncoms barely slept before having to get back on the trail to join their comrades.

Back in Midhar, Jens and most of the other nurses found themselves wedged into a tiny home that doubled as the shelter for the family's goats. The women had to pick up a sleeping baby goat to find enough room for everyone to stretch out.

Their feet ached from the day's exertions; there was no food available, but they were so pooped they would have fallen asleep in seconds. But the little goat kept licking Jens's toes. Jens would nudge it away with her foot—but that only encouraged the animal. Finally, their hostess got up and dragged the kid by the nape of the neck, hugging it next to her so it wouldn't bother the visitors.

No one got any decent rest. They were cold and miserable, overcome by anxiety and diarrhea.

After a few scant hours, the nurses told Duffy they wanted to get rolling.

"After so many reversals," Jens wrote, "[we] were obsessed with getting to the coast before anything else happened. 'The Coast' became the magic word for all kinds of help."

There was no more codeine or morphine available, so there was little they could do to dull the ache of their infirmities. Better to push on to the Adriatic than sit around pining for rest, food, and medication that would never come.

Their goal on January 5 was Golem. Part of the trail they would take that day they'd been on before, heading the other way. They knew it would be rough going.

But the weather made things worse. A pounding rain, complete with thunder and lightning, tormented them all day. They passed the carcass of a dead mule that morning and hoped it wasn't an omen. The afternoon rain turned to sleet, then hail. They couldn't wait to get to Golem, where Duffy thought there was a decent chance a meal could be arranged.

Nurse Tacina's ankles began to swell that morning. She kept refusing to be placed on a mule until Duffy issued one of his don't-screw-with-me directives. By the time Tassy climbed onto the donkey, her ankles were blue, swollen to twice their normal size.

Steffa and Thrasher were waiting for them in Golem when the group arrived at about 1300. The two scouts were pleasantly surprised that the larger party was running hours ahead of schedule. It was the third time in recent days that the Americans had passed through Golem, which caused a few of them to spew profanities. The people of Golem were no doubt as tired of seeing the Americans as the Americans were of trudging through Golem.

They were again divided by gender and rank, with the noncoms forced to bunk in a house that was a long slog up the mountain. But their hosts fed them an edible meal, which they fell on "like savages," Abbot wrote, "every man for himself, and cleaning up the pot and grumbling for more."

In his report filed from Golem, Duffy noted that certain members of the party were on the verge of cracking up—and he wasn't far off himself. They had pulled into Golem in the middle of a hailstorm, "looking like a bunch of prisoners on the Russian front," he wrote.

They were having a "rough time in this area," Duffy told his superiors. It would be essential, he stressed, for the group to have food and shelter waiting for them when they reached the seaside.

The good news was that if the latest reports were accurate, Captain Lloyd Smith should have been getting close to their position.

It turned out that Smith had, through some well-connected Partisans, expropriated a truck. Smith's entourage coaxed and bribed its way through BK territory, pulling into the village of Vuno at about nine o'clock the night of the fifth. A month into his quest, he was finally within reach of his goal.

FINAL DASH
TO FREEDOM

•

January 6–9, 1944

Drino River

YUGOSLAVIA

Port Wilson

MACEDONIA

Adriatic Sea

ALBANIA

Vjosë River

AREA OF DETAIL

GREECE

Ionian Sea

Vlorë

Vjosë River

to Bari

Seaview (pickup location)

Dukat

Terbaci

Gramma Bay
(Sea Elephant)

Mount Dukati

Kalarat

Kuç

Llongora Pass

Dhermi

Golem

Vuno

Ionian Sea

| 0 | Miles | 10 | 20 |

| 0 | Kilometers | 20 |

© 2013 Jeffrey L. Ward

The weather turned even uglier the next morning, January 6. An icy blanket of snow covered the ground, causing the mules to get colicky. Only after repeated kicks from the guides did the animals cooperate.

They had to scale a mountain that morning; the slush underfoot would make the task tougher. Tacina was still bothered by sore ankles. When just fifty yards out she keeled over, Duffy ordered her back onto the mule.

The snow turned into a blizzard so intense that their lead guide got disoriented, heading them in the wrong direction for thirty minutes. That night, Duffy reported to his bosses that the snow was so heavy you couldn't see your hand in front of your face. Furious that they'd taken a wrong turn, Duffy lit into the guide.

"For the first time," the British lieutenant wrote, "I lost my temper and nearly strangled him; at the same time, my interpreter conveyed verbally my wish. We then set off again and after an hour, passed out of the blizzard. How the girls took it, I do not know."

Not only the "girls" but the "boys," too, couldn't help but think that being on top of a mountain in the middle of a blizzard was déjà vu of which they wanted no part. Abbott again found himself groping along a slippery mountain trace, eyes almost blinded, trying to follow an indistinguishable mass in front of him.

Their guides were mumbling something that sounded to Abbott like a talismanic hymn, praying for good luck as they stumbled toward the summit.

The Albanians sang it low and rhythmically, among themselves, but the Americans all hoped their Tosk obeisance to the snow gods would rub off. It did—until one of the women, "Miss Tacina," as Duffy called her in his report, nearly met her maker. The mule on which Tassy was riding lost its footing, even though Duffy was holding on to its tail, Albanian-style, as they inched down the mountain. Tassy pitched forward, tumbling toward a drop of some fifteen feet that could have killed her. Duffy made a headlong dive and caught hold of her belt in the nick of time.

"We both rolled down the hill together," he wrote, "emerging from the drift, just two huge snow balls! Luckily, neither one of us was hurt."

It was a minor miracle that Tassy's spill did not aggravate her injury. It was also near-miraculous that no one broke an ankle or seriously wrenched a knee in their two-month ordeal. A disabling injury to any of them would have proven disastrous.

The mules had not been fed for two days, Duffy reported, and were beginning to break down. Still, the group pushed on, now gunning for Kuç and, beyond it, Kalarat—and somewhere in there, a hoped-for rendezvous with the OSS captain, food, and rest.

They trudged forward at a snail's pace, braving conditions almost as vexing as any they had experienced, Abbott recalled. Every step demanded such concentration that they became almost oblivious to the wet and cold.

Inevitably, there were two more crossings of Devoll tributaries. The first waterway was fairly narrow; the guides led the group across a series of stepping-stones. Duffy and Blondie, wearing thick rubber boots, helped sling the nurses from stone to stone, which wasn't an easy task for the women with shorter legs.

Bill Eldridge elicited howls when he took a running leap toward the first stone, slipped, and collapsed into the water. He came up cursing a blue streak, which culminated with "G-g-go t-t-to h-h-hell!" Beyond a bruised ego, he emerged unhurt, as did the rest of the gang.

On her last stepping-stone, however, Tooie Dawson overcompensated, jumping too far. Duffy, trying to catch her, lost his balance, too. In his report that night, he described Dawson as coming at him "like a tornado." The two of them careered into thigh-deep water, with Duffy getting the worst of it.

He helped pulled Dawson out, then grabbed his wayward

tommy gun and "strode off down the trail without a word or backward glance," Abbott remembered. "He was so mad you could almost see his clothes steaming."

No one's clothes steamed on the second crossing. The guides discovered a bridge downstream, which enabled them to get to Kuç ahead of schedule, around three o'clock that afternoon.

Duffy immediately dispatched the guides to question villagers about the whereabouts of Captain Smith. No one had seen or heard about an American officer, so they shoved on.

Only a half hour elapsed before they bumped into a heavyset Caucasian with a blond beard hiking toward them. He was sporting a British military coat over his mackinaw and carrying a long walking stick. As he got closer, the Americans realized he was wearing paratrooper's boots and a U.S. Army cap.

CHAPTER 10

FINAL DASH TO FREEDOM

"My God, it's Smith, Captain Smith, that is!" Jens exclaimed as the stocky figure grew closer.

As they welcomed him with handshakes and back thumps, Smith grinned and said that he hadn't been expecting to see them for another day or two. Duffy grinned back and told him the group had, despite everything, been making damn good time.

His fellow Americans told Smith that they'd heard rumors he'd been captured by the enemy three weeks earlier. The captain responded by saying that he'd heard the same scuttlebutt about them, reinforcing Duffy's view that a soldier can never believe hearsay rattling around a war zone.

They gave Smith a rapid-fire rundown on what had happened to them in recent weeks, then listened as he shared what he knew about their situation from intelligence reports, and his plan to get them to the coast.

The airmen in the rescue armada, Smith reported, were convinced that the castaways had been killed in Gjirokastër—all but Major McKnight, who insisted that they were still safe and wanted to mount another rescue effort right away. For the December 29 attempt, McKnight had squirreled away on his C-47 a "whole PX-full of cigarettes, candy, chewing gum, drinks, food, medicines and everything else" they could possibly need.

When Smith shared the news that the P-38s returning from the aborted rescue had annihilated an enemy truck convoy, the Americans exulted. McKnight's cargo plane had absorbed some flak damage, but had returned to Bari safely.

He also shared the remarkable revelation that the 807th's plight had become "grapevine news" all through the Mediterranean theater. "We've all but been at war with British intelligence because all the dope we've had was just what they wanted to tell us," Smith said, to Duffy's amusement.

"The day you get back," Smith said, chortling, "the news wires [will] be plenty hot, only I've a hunch they're going to keep you bottled up for a while."

It would be okay by him, Paul Allen joked, if they stayed bottled up indefinitely.

Smith then explained that he had been trained to help Tito's Partisans in Yugoslavia but had been temporarily assigned to Albania once the C-53 went down. The captain asked when they'd heard last from or about the three other nurses in Berat. When told they had heard nothing, Smith acknowledged that the OSS was also in the dark. The SOE had devised a plan to get them out, but Smith had no information as to where it all stood.

Duffy volunteered that in his estimation the nurses in Berat had to be safe.

Why so confident? Smith asked his counterpart.

"Unless the Germans have changed their tactics, they're more inclined to spout that kind of news than we are," Duffy replied. "And there hasn't been a word from anywhere. [The Germans] haven't even spun any fairy tales about them."

How could Allied intelligence get to Maness, Lytle, and Porter? the Americans asked. With a combination of bribery and bravado, there might be a chance of sneaking a vehicle through checkpoints and motoring to the sea, the officers said.

Jens recalled the acerbic McKenzie piping up, "Wouldn't that beat all, if they get a ride to the coast while we have climbed, slipped, and slid all over this country for sixty days?"

There was no time for further pleasantries. Smith and Duffy said they had to get back on the trail to Kalarat. As they readied themselves to leave, Smith imparted good news: After more than a week of occupation, the Germans had evacuated Terbaci, opening a more direct route for the Americans to get to the Adriatic.

Had the enemy stayed in Terbaci, the group would have been forced to climb an additional mountain range. Smith said he had hidden provisions in a cavern southwest of the village of Palasa in the event that they would have to head that direction. It would have taken four full days to reach the coastal base had they been forced to sidestep Terbaci. Now if everything fell into place, they could do it in three days, possibly fewer, Smith said.

It took three hours of arduous hiking to get to Kalarat that night. Smith's largesse produced the desired results: Food and shelter were quickly arranged despite the lateness of the hour.

Steffa had desperately wanted to escape with the Americans to Italy. But his eleventh-hour pleadings with Duffy and Smith apparently went unheeded. At dawn on the morning of

January 7, Steffa said good-bye, explaining that there were too many BK fighters and German troops between Kalarat and the sea.

Jens and the others were guilt-ridden that they had ever doubted his loyalties—although he had given them plenty of seeds to sow those misgivings. Steffa reminded Jens that he had two brothers in Cleveland, Ohio, and asked her to look them up and assure them that Steffa and his family were getting along "in spite of everything."

She promised to track down his siblings, reminding him that one of her nicest moments in Albania had been playing cards with Steffa's mother in Berat. He was wiping away tears as Jens took off her flight wings and pressed them into his hands, telling him she wanted Steffa's son Alfredo to have them.

"He'll be very pleased. I remember how excited he was because he thought you were a pilot," Steffa told her as they both laughed. They shook hands a second time as Jens thanked him for everything he'd done.

Steffa's farewell with the noncoms was less emotional. Abbott remembered Steffa maintaining that he had to leave with Pandee because he didn't trust the guide to communicate the correct message back to the Partisan leadership. If Pandee's message could be construed that Steffa had somehow deserted the Partisan cause, his wife and children might be murdered, he said. It was yet another head-scratching statement from someone who'd been making them for seven weeks.

Abbott remembered Thrasher and Baggs giving Steffa their tommy guns and ammunition, plus emptying their pockets of what little Albanian coin they had left.

"I suppose we have to admit he had earned it and more," Abbott wrote. "But that Steffa! Even now, we all wondered if he wasn't skipping out because he didn't like our chances of getting through on this last lap."

Steffa's parting gesture was to pull out a handkerchief, blow his nose, and declaim, "You have now not a very long way to go."

With Pandee leaving, too, the Americans worried about the caliber of the remaining guides on their final push to the coast. They observed two men aligned with Smith helping get everyone organized. The men's loyalty to Smith had, in all probability, been purchased. But the Americans could be forgiven for fearing that the scouts weren't exactly devoted to the Allied cause.

They got under way at dawn, heading toward Seaview, the SOE embarkation point situated another dozen miles or more northwest. Many in the party turned to wave at Steffa and Pandee, departing at the same time. Eventually the pair disappeared, meandering up a northern trail.

Jens looked at the name and address on the scrap of paper that Steffa had given her. If it ever fell into enemy hands, it would be damning. The Gestapo could easily trace it to Steffa and his family in Berat. She transferred a part of the address to one section of her barely legible "diary," then scribbled the rest in another section, hoping the Germans would not be able to draw the connection. Then she tore Steffa's note into tiny pieces and tossed them into the brush at different points on the trail.

Early that morning, they had to cross a stream, most likely the River Shushica. Willis Shumway, sore knee and all, ferried the nurses, piggybacking them through nearly waist-deep water. Duffy, Smith, Blondie, Willie, and the guides eyeballed the surrounding hills for signs of hostile activity. None was spotted.

The two special ops officers had made it plain that soon the group would be entering territory dominated by the BK; the Balli leaders were in league with the Nazis, but Smith had made certain "arrangements" to secure the party's safety. Abbott referred to this new territory as "Barley Corn Tar" turf. The last of the Partisan fighters guiding them at Duffy's direction left the party as it reached the summit of a large hill; with so many unfriendlies on the other side, it was too hazardous for him to continue.

"There would be undercover Patriots, havens here and there along the way," Abbott wrote, "but aside from these, we had to count everyone as hostile, or at least owing us no loyalty or friendship."

Barleys notwithstanding, the group wanted to push west, no matter the risk. When they stopped for a few minutes' break, one of the mule drivers said his animals were too ground down and would have to turn back.

"It was plain that [the mule driver] thought we were heading into certain trouble and he wanted no part of it," Abbott recalled. "At last, the native simply turned his back on Smith and started to walk away. He had taken only a few steps when the captain snapped out a word in Albanian. The mule driver froze in his tracks, and then turned slowly to face the .45 service automatic held steady as a rock in Smith's right fist.

"The eyes of the two met for a moment. Then, without a word, the American made a peremptory motion with the gun towards the mules. The driver moved sullenly over to his place in the caravan. Smith, gun still in hand, watched them set off, the loads swaying with the stride of the beasts and the heads of the men, outlined sharp and black against the twilight sky, bobbing into cadence to their mountain gait. Smith shoved the gun slowly into its holster. He spoke without turning his head to us.

"'Let's go now,' he said, quietly."

Smith knew that back in Bari a special boat was primed at a moment's notice to cross the Strait of Otranto to pick up the group at Seaview. The name of the launch was *Yankee*; its skipper was a freewheeling Marine lieutenant on interim assignment with the OSS. The skipper's gift for special ops and negotiating tough waters—literally and figuratively—had made him a coveted commodity in the Mediterranean theater. The leathery-faced leatherneck's nom de guerre was John Hamilton; his real-life name, though, was Sterling Hayden. In his wayward youth, Hayden had abandoned prep school to sail the world on a schooner and dabble now and again in acting.

He found his way to Hollywood in the late thirties. Just before Pearl Harbor, Hayden had shown promise as a B-movie tough guy, starring in low-budget film noirs. Once America entered the war, he joined the Marines and was eventually sent to OSS's Mediterranean operations. Clandestine missions in the MTO depended in no small measure on pinpoint boat landings, often carried out under the cloak of darkness. Hamilton/Hayden was the perfect man for the job: The taciturn Marine knew how to operate a boat in choppy water and feather an engine without being detected.

Hamilton was living the sort of grizzled man-against-the-world role for which he would become celebrated in pictures such as *The Asphalt Jungle* and, much later, *The Godfather*, where his character, the corrupt police captain, would be subjected to one of the grisliest murders in film history.

Naar got to know Hamilton in Bari. "He rarely spoke to anyone," Naar says today, but the American actor must have enjoyed the company of the iconoclastic Brit. Over beers at Bari's Imperiale Hotel, Naar grew to admire the Yank, who seemed to be waging his own private war. Hamilton was that rare American who not only understood what SOE was trying to accomplish but wanted to work in tandem with the Brits. Like Naar, Quayle, and Tilman, he was also not unsympathetic to the Partisans' political leanings.

Hamilton and his *Yankee* crew were put on alert December 8 and told not to leave Bari. At any moment they might be needed to fetch Lloyd Smith or ferry the American refugees back across the strait.

No doubt Hamilton and his men had joined in cleaning up the mess that was Bari Harbor. On December 2, 1943, three weeks after the C-53's crash-landing in Albania, more than a hundred German Ju 88 bombers of Luftflotte 2 based in northern Italy pummeled Bari and its harbor, inflicting hundreds of casualties. Twenty-seven Allied cargo and transport ships were sunk or damaged—but fortunately for the stranded Americans, Hamilton's *Yankee* was not among them.

Some historians call the attack on Bari "the Little Pearl Harbor." For reasons never fully explained, one of the British ships destroyed in the harbor was carrying poisonous mustard gas, apparently as a contingency if Hitler resorted to the use of chemical weapons in the Mediterranean. The toxin spread all over Bari, exacting more casualties and rendering the harbor unusable for days. Both during and after the war, the Allies suppressed information about the horrendous fallout from the Bari bombing.

The 807th's remaining nurses and medics in Catania joined other MAES units in rushing to Bari to tend to the sick and wounded.

As the party pushed toward Terbaci on January 7, the weather turned even tougher. Jens recalled one mule after another collapsing in deep snow, with some of the taller men pushing ahead to break a path. Still, neither a blizzard nor darkness deterred them.

They finally reached Dukat around midnight. Here Smith's palm-greasing began to pay big dividends. He and his men had done their advance work, spreading cash in the right places. Despite the lateness of the hour, several homes immediately opened their doors, with Smith and his guides shooing the refugees inside.

The nurses were ushered into the best-appointed home they'd seen on their travels. They didn't know it, but they were probably in a dwelling owned by Isuf Shehaj, an associate of Xheli Çela, the local BK chieftain who was the most powerful man in southwestern Albania.

Tea was served to them on an ornate tray. The American women peeked inside a bowl. It was too good to be true: sugar, practically their first taste of it since they'd left Catania two months before. They all put extra dollops into their tea and tore into dainty pastries, corn bread cakes, and goat cheese. Admiring the family's belongings, the ladies concluded that the home must have belonged to landed gentry, not the sort of Albanians likely to be supporting a peasants' insurrection. They wondered how Smith had managed to pull off such a coup but were too tired—and polite—to ask pointed questions.

But the real surprise was waiting for them when they emerged from the house a few minutes later. An old Italian army truck was sitting on Dukat's only street.

Captain Smith stood at the back of the truck and spoke quietly but forcefully. He said the Germans controlled the road they'd be taking; at any minute, they could expect enemy patrols to pounce. If forced to abandon the truck, they should head toward the nearest peak in the Dukati mountain range due west; if somehow they got separated and were being pursued, everyone should plan to climb over the summit. Once they reached the far side, they wouldn't be far from the sea.

Smith also said that if he, Duffy, Blondie, Williamson, and another British soldier who had joined them from Seaview named Bert—all armed with machine guns—were forced to use firearms, they would make quick work of the enemy. If the group heard gunfire, everyone was to flatten themselves, then take deeper cover.

They crowded into the back of the truck, almost afraid to

breathe. A mile or so outside Dukat, the vehicle abruptly stopped. Smith assured them that everything was fine. Two shadowy figures emerged from the woods, each carrying a canister of gasoline. They poured the fuel into the truck's tank before vanishing.

The truck "growled and wheezed down the road," Abbott remembered. Every time it hit a pothole, the lorry lurched, jostling its occupants.

They'd been in the truck for about half an hour when Smith suddenly ordered them out. He'd spotted headlights bearing toward them and had to assume it was a German patrol car.

"Everybody get out! Get into the brush, but fast!" Smith yelled.

They needed no urging, Abbott recalled. "We scrambled out of there. I ducked into the bushes on the run and went forty yards up the slope until I brought up a patch of briars where I found Mac-Kinnon. All around we could hear the rustle of other groups."

Paula Kanable, cursing a blue streak, as was her wont, complained that she'd been trampled by "elephants."

"Next time," she snarled, "I'll let the sons of bitches go and just stay on the truck."

Jens reported that a male voice said with a cackle, "Can we depend on that?"

Abbott heard Paul Allen mumble an oath about losing his hat. Duffy bleated, "Stay right where you are and keep your blooming mouth shut!"

They kept their mouths shut and waited, hearts pounding, for an enemy vehicle to appear. None did.

The group piled back into the truck. After only a hundred yards, though, they heard Smith yell, "Stop!"

Dead ahead, he had spotted the black outline of another vehicle parked on the side of the road.

"If they snap on their lights," Smith ordered, "hit the bush!"

Standing outside the driver's door, Smith quickly reviewed

options with Duffy and the Albanian driver. With that, the driver cautiously began striding toward the stalled vehicle.

"We watched him go," Abbott wrote, "and I don't think there was anybody who would have traded shoes with him right then. The man moved perhaps ten paces out in front of our truck. With the suddenness of a whack of a club the road leaped into a glare of light."

Everyone dived out the back of the truck, with various invocations of "Jesus!" being made through bated breath. Abbott felt like a scared jackrabbit as he tore into the woods. They all believed that shots would ring out and they'd be dead.

"By the feel of it, the hair on my head was standing straight up," Abbott wrote.

They kept waiting, but nothing happened. From their spot in the trees they watched Smith confer with the Albanian driver.

"All aboard! Come on!" Smith yelled. "We're getting out of here!"

It turned out the parked vehicle was indeed a German truck, but it had been stolen by a pair of Partisans who were trying to drive it toward friendlier territory. On their end, the armed thieves had assumed the opposing group was a German patrol. Everyone was lucky there hadn't been an exchange of panicky gunfire.

The getaway truck resumed its wheezing. For mile after mile, they staggered down the road, amazed that no other set of headlights came over either horizon. By now it was two hours or more past midnight.

They came to a noisy halt in front of a farmhouse set a distance from the road. "All off," Smith ordered.

The group shuffled up what Abbott described as a well-worn path to the house. Their truck driver pulled off the main road and concealed the vehicle. As the group reached the house, they spotted headlights a mile or so down the road.

"Nobody had to ask any questions about this car," Abbott wrote. "It fairly yelled Nazi patrol from the moment it came in sight until both the sound and lights had faded into the distance. We let our breaths go in a sigh of relief."

The farmhouse belonged to people—most likely Çela associates and BK sympathizers—who, with Smith's coin in their pockets, fed them and let them rest for an hour or so. At Smith's urging, they left their equipment at the house; it would catch up to them later, he promised.

They were back on foot, hiking up Dukati Mountain, the last barrier to the coast. At dawn, several hours later, they were still on the narrow trail, stumbling toward the summit. Smith and Duffy called frequent rest stops; each time, the Americans would urge the leaders to get cracking.

At around nine o'clock on the morning of the eighth they finally crested the snowcapped summit of Dukati Mountain.

"There, in broad daylight ahead of us, was the sea!" Abbott enthused. "Sight of it almost overpowered us for a minute. We simply stood and stared at that patch of open water."

Irishman Jim Cruise spoke for all of them when he said, "God bless us all this blessed, blessed day."

Jens heard someone gasp, "We made it! I knew we could. I just knew we'd make it!" She looked around to see who'd said it before realizing it had come out of her own mouth.

Duffy and Smith left little time for prayerful gaping. The caravan still had to slither past enemy strongholds and patrols.

With adrenaline now surging, they worked their way down the hill. It was a surprisingly easy descent; there were few obstacles and no enemy-occupied settlements to sidestep.

At about one o'clock in the afternoon they reached the foot of the mountain, where SOE operatives from Seaview greeted them with American cigarettes and candy bars. There Blondie and Williamson beamed a radio message across the strait to Bari. A while later they got a flash back: Lieutenant Hamilton's *Yankee* would be off the shore around midnight that night to pick them up. In a daze, now escorted by a British patrol, they stumbled toward Seaview.

They were amazed by Seaview's warren of caves. Smith led them to the main cavern. A shiny gray rock sat in the middle. SOE and OSS had supplied the hideaway with food and blankets and eight or ten crude cots. They ate a little—Jens remembered an OSS officer scrambling some eggs—but slept fitfully. Jens was so sick and exhausted, though, she collapsed. Most kept looking outside, praying that darkness would descend. Finally, it did.

Duffy and Smith had hiked down to the shoreline to pin down logistical arrangements for the *Yankee*'s arrival and quick departure. A rowboat would take members of the party out to the waiting launch in groups of three or four.

"No lights, no smoking, and keep your talk low," Smith told those still awake.

They dozed on and off. The tension was unbearable. Finally, just after midnight there was a flicker of light out on the water.

"That's her!" Abbott stage-whispered. "She's my baby!"

Garry came striding up, "his boots grinding in the sandy gravel," Abbott remembered. "All right, you chaps, get ready to load," Duffy said. "That's our bally boat out there." They didn't need to be told twice.

Jens was still sleeping when someone shook her awake.

"Jens. Jensen, wake up! Come on, get up! Come on; the boat is here!"

By the time Jens got down to the shoreline, two groups had already been rowed out. It was so dark it was hard to tell, but the *Yankee* did not appear to be overly sleek. In fact, once they got closer, the launch looked like an elongated tugboat, with an unseemly pilothouse sprouting out of its deck like a snout. But it must have seemed gorgeous to them. It moved fast enough over open water;

Hamilton knew how to steer the ugly duckling around enemy naval patrols.

It stayed deathly quiet onshore. When it was finally Jens's turn, four other members of the party joined her as SOE men and Albanian guides shoved the rowboat out to sea. It pitched in the wintertime waves. Bitterly cold water spilled in, drenching their shoes and pant legs.

It took almost fifteen minutes, but at last they reached the *Yankee*. A tall man in a black overcoat, quite possibly the noir movie king in the flesh, tossed down a rope ladder and said, "Crawl up. Hold the ropes tight!"

He and another crewman reached down and helped Jens and the others climb aboard. They kept their viselike grip on Jens as they walked her across the unlighted deck and down four steps to the cabin, where pillows and blankets—and abundant amounts of rum and candy—awaited.

The crew members were surprised that Jens and the others could walk with little exertion. From what they'd been told, the Americans would be in pitiful physical shape.

A series of dull lanterns illuminated the cabin. Jens could hear American and British voices topside, quietly jabbering.

She didn't want to listen: All she wanted to do was hit the head, slip underneath a blanket, and go back to sleep. But Ann Markowitz, who'd been on board for a while, was hugging the porcelain toilet, moaning.

Jens was worried that Marky had tripped and hurt herself, but it turned out she was just violently seasick. Since Jens needed to use the commode, Marky moved away, but not before commenting that the water closet was "beautiful" and "so white!" Having spent two months puking and defecating in the great Albanian outdoors, it was a thrill for them to use a Western commode.

Within minutes they felt a powerful surge. They were heading toward Italy.

"After that we simply concentrated on taking it easy," Abbott wrote. "We were too worn-out to get much of a kick out of the greatest of all miracles, we were really going home! We were out of Albania; free at last from the threat of Jerries; and all we wanted was a hundred years of rest."

They spent the rest of the night in a stupor, fueled in part by the rum the crew was now liberally dispensing. The crew told them in midvoyage that a naval skirmish between Allied and German boats had broken out due west; the *Yankee* had to sweep south to avoid getting caught in it. A few hours off the Italian coast the sea became extremely rough; several of them, Abbott included, began upchucking.

"By that time those of us who were poor sailors wouldn't have given a damn if our course had taken us through action between the combined fleets," Abbott remembered. The medics for the most part hung up on deck while the nurses rested below. But when land was sighted, everyone tumbled topside, seasickness be cursed. They motored past the seaside villas of Brindisi as they made their way toward Bari.

At about 1330, the *Yankee* pulled into Bari Harbor. They ran below to grab the musette bags they'd dragged across half the mountains in Albania. Most of the nurses brushed their hair, splashed water on their faces, and used whatever lipstick and powder they could find to make themselves a bit more presentable. It had taken them a half day to get across the strait.

They all gathered at the rail to wave at the astonishingly large crowd that had gathered on the dock. Fifty-eight days removed, it was their welcome to Berat redux. As the *Yankee* drew closer, they realized the redheaded officer standing on the dock was none other than Major McKnight, the 807th's boss.

"There's the Old Man!" they yelped, touched that he had come down to the pier to welcome them home. It had been twelve days since McKnight had packed a C-47 transport full of cigarettes and chocolates. Now Red was able to dispense his goodies without worrying about being peppered by German artillery.

Captain Robert Simpson, the officer who, sixty-two days earlier, facetiously asked whether anyone had "any last words" as the C-53 revved up in Catania, was on the dock, too. So were a flock of U.S. intelligence officers and what appeared to Duffy to be a small army of still photographers and at least one film cameraman.

Jon Naar and his SOE colleagues in B8 were on the pier, too, ready to congratulate Duffy, Bell, and Williamson on a job well-done. There was practically one photographer for every nurse in the party, Naar remembered, an object lesson in the U.S. preoccupation with flash and dazzle.

"For us Brits," Naar wrote, "it was an illuminating lesson in the then-new art of Public Relations—putting the most positive face on the conduct of war in conformity with the underlying political ends our leaders had in mind rather than with what really had taken place."

The whole scene was bizarre. One minute the escapees were seasick, thrilled to be puking over a rail instead of into an Albanian bush; the next they were making their way up a ramp, engulfed by VIPs and photographers. Behind the knot of people were spanking-new American sedans, lined up to cruise them to the 26th General Hospital. The facility was literally brand-new, having been hastily constructed after Bari's December 2 bombing.

The Americans, Lloyd Smith included, were ushered into the staff cars, while the Brits, the Yanks' protectors for several hundred miles through enemy territory—Lieutenant Duffy, Sergeant Bell, and Corporal Williamson—were relegated to a heap that Naar's team had driven out to the air base. Without fanfare and flashing bulbs, the Brits were driven to SOE's headquarters in Bari, where they were debriefed before heading out to the Imperiale Hotel bar for a few glasses of "plonk"—Tommy slang for cheap wine.

In the Brits' minds, much of the episode had been a gigantic snafu (in their argot, "semi-non-adjustable fuck up"), punctuated by the biggest fuckup of all—Washington's insistence on a quixotic attempt at an air rescue. Still, even the Brits had to admit, with characteristic understatement, that things had worked out more or less okay.

Even before they could rid themselves of their lice-infested clothes, the Americans were interrogated by U.S. G-2 intelligence officers. The two pilots were whisked away for special questioning and were not seen again by the others. A major who questioned Jens wanted to know precisely what villages they had trekked through and who among the Partisans had been of greatest assistance.

Jens pulled out her diary scribbles to help jog her memory of where the group had been and how they had gotten there. The major immediately commandeered her notes, saying, "I'll have to take those."

When Jens protested, he assured her that she could get them back someday by writing to the Prisoner of War Department in Washington, D.C. Decades later, when she submitted her request, she was amazed that the diary, completely intact, was mailed to her.

During the debriefing, she happened to praise the reputation of Harry Fultz, the American teacher who had mentored Steffa and Hasan at the school operated by the American Red Cross. The major perfunctorily nodded, then said, "As long as you are in this theater, don't mention his name again." She had no way of knowing that Fultz, while still technically a "civilian," was a key OSS Balkans strategist.

They were all given stern warnings that divulging particulars of their ordeal might compromise Albania's Partisan network and the integrity of Allied resistance operations. At various points in the coming days and weeks, they were all forced to sign nondisclosure documents. Harold Hayes remembers signing four separate promissories.

OSS and SOE didn't want the Germans to know the efficacy of the Allied special ops apparatus in Eastern Europe or the Balkans. And now that Hitler was on the run, the U.S., especially, did not want favorable publicity fawned on Hoxha, Tito, or Stalin, even though, as Naar points out, the Red Air Force had become an increasingly potent force in the MTO.

With all that vodka drinking, the Bari-based pilots had helped immeasurably improve Naar's Russian.

USAAF public relations arranged for Associated Press columnist Harold V. "Hal" Boyle to cover the Bari homecoming. Boyle was an effusive second-generation Irishman from Kansas City whose syndicated column, "Leaves from a War Correspondent's Notebook," was second in popularity only to the writings of Ernie Pyle. Hal was well equipped to recount the 807th's odyssey: He had a shanachie's gift for feature writing, loved extolling the derring-do of ordinary Americans, and adored everything about women. Boyle must have spent a day or two in Bari, interviewing the principals and getting briefed by public relations officers.

Boyle's AP story ended up being sat on for more than a month: It didn't clear censors and appear in U.S. papers, among them the *Atlanta Constitution*, the *Hartford Courant*, and the *Baltimore Sun*, until mid-February. Boyle was deliberately fed a ton of misleading information. The Brits got nary a mention in Boyle's piece, he paid only lip service to the bravery of the Albanian Partisans, and his chronology of the ordeal was all mixed-up. Everything had to be written in code to keep the enemy at bay, of course, but military officials should have ensured that more of Boyle's facts bore some semblance of reality.

The hospital was so new that the Albanian escapees were its first patients. They all got warm baths, matching dark robes, and pajamas and slippers that did not have little animals crawling around in them.

Jens's fears about Jim Cruise's health were borne out: He was diagnosed with walking pneumonia and confined to bed for two weeks. Doctors also fretted about a boil they found on Jens's ankle and insisted that she, too, stay in bed. She needed the rest: Her stomach was distended and her intestinal system was a mess. Within days, their personal stuff arrived from Catania, so they were able to put on some familiar clothes.

At some point early on, the nurses agreed to pose for a series of photographs for public consumption. The pictures in Jens's scrapbook are inscribed, "January 9, 1944," but judging from how good their hair and makeup looked, it's a safe bet the photo shoot took place a while after the *Yankee* pulled into Bari.

Pauleen Kanable, the onetime airline hostess who seven weeks earlier had calmly dabbed on lipstick as a Nazi tank menaced them outside Berat, looked especially glamorous. She had painted her nails red but must not have been pleased with how her hair looked that day. Paula kept her tresses under a flight cap and was the only one wearing a hat for the occasion. Fran Nelson donned a fetching white scarf.

No doubt at the direction of a USAAF public relations officer, the nurses buttoned on their tattered (but presumably cleaned-up) uniforms and laced up their beat-up boots. Paula, Lillian Tacina, and Ann Kopsco all wore their trench coats; the others wore shorter "Eisenhower jackets" that were almost definitely not part of their Albanian wardrobe, unless they had been parachuted in late in the game by the Brits.

The best shot taken that day was of six of them laughing as they pointed out that their boot soles had been worn almost through.

When, five weeks later, Army censors finally allowed the story and photos to clear, it was the boot-bottom picture that got the widest play back home. Someone familiar with Albania's topography estimated that by the time they reached Seaview, the Americans had trekked some seven or eight hundred miles up and around Albania. No wonder their boot soles were shot.

All thirteen medics, plus noncoms Shumway and Lebo, had their pictures taken in matching robes, gathered around the bedridden Cruise, whose head was propped up by a pair of pillows. Separately, the ten nurses were also pictured in their robes, their hair and makeup by that point impeccable. A charming photograph was taken of Duffy being simultaneously kissed by two nurses—Lillian Tacina was bussing one cheek and Fran Nelson the other.

By coincidence, OSS head Bill Donovan and his SOE counterpart, Major-General Sir Colin McVean Gubbins, happened to be in Bari on official duty that week. Donovan went out of his way to greet the freed Americans, even checking up on Jens and other nurses a couple of days later in the hospital.

Jon Naar watched Donovan commend Duffy for going above and beyond the call of duty. After weeks of not-so-veiled threats against the Brits, the OSS leader relayed FDR's personal appreciation for SOE's efforts in springing the Yanks from Albania.

Jens spent twelve days in the Bari hospital before being allowed to rejoin the 807th in Catania. In World War II, the U.S. military had a hard-and-fast rule: No soldier who escaped after an extended period behind enemy lines could remain in that battle theater. If they had stayed in the Mediterranean and been captured, the members of the 807th and their airmen could have been accused by the Germans of perpetrating espionage. Each member was given an extended leave back in the States while officials tried to figure out their next assignments.

Orville Abbott, Bob Owen, Paul Allen, and Charlie Adams hitched a plane ride from Catania to Oran, then to Gibraltar, Rabat, and Casablanca, where they were forced to cool their heels for a few days while waiting for a transatlantic flight to come open.

They were having beers in Casablanca one night when they happened to bump into a B-25 pilot with the 12th Army Air Force. Swapping war stories, they shared their Albanian trauma. The bomber jock smiled and said he'd been part of a raid on the Berat airport in November.

"Did they smoke one of your ships?" Abbott's gang asked the pilot.

"I'll say," the pilot answered. "Mine."

"I'll be damned," Abbott remarked.

Less than two years later, Abbott was to write, "We sat a moment in silence. For all of us, there was again the sight of those roaring, speeding planes over our heads on that day so far, far away now. We heard again the crump of their bombs on the Nazi field. We felt the sink of our hearts at the plume of black smoke streaming from one of the ships."

"'Guess we prayed you back,' Owen mused. The flyer met Bob's eyes.

"'We were doing some ourselves,' he said. 'But thanks for the support.'"

Lieutenant Agnes Jensen began her journey back home to Michigan on January 23, 1944—seventy-four days after the C-53 took off from Catania. When she finally arrived at the farm in Stanwood, she learned that her parents had been informed via telegram that she was alive, and not in enemy hands, right around her twenty-ninth birthday in early December. Her folks forgave her for not mentioning that she'd volunteered for flight evacuation duty.

She got a three-week furlough before having to report back to Bowman Field in Louisville. Once back at Bowman she joined fellow 807th nurse Jean Rutkowski in becoming a senior instructor in the flight nurse trainer program. Among other subjects, they taught emergency training; given their experience, they had no trouble getting their pupils' attention. One of Jens's regular duties was to accompany nurses and medics on their first missions to pick up wounded warriors from airfields around the country, helping trainees overcome their apprehensions.

That spring, Jens was asked to participate in a cross-country war bond drive along with other heroic veterans. A C-47 cargo plane was requisitioned to fly the bond team around the country. In the middle of their tour, a mind-boggling scenario transpired: The transport experienced engine trouble. Its pilot was forced to pull off an emergency landing on a civilian crop-duster strip in northwestern Iowa, outside a village called Spirit Lake. The strip proved too short for the C-47; the plane careened off the end of the runway, its nose crumpling against a tree. Miraculously, no one was hurt.

For the second time in less than a year, Jens had survived a hair-raising crash-landing—but this one was mild compared to her experience in Albania. At least around Spirit Lake there weren't Nazi patrols lurking or men with thick mustaches and red-starred hats hugging her—and calling her a savior.

CHAPTER 11

RESCUING THE MISSING THREE

OSS liked to give colorful code names to each of its clandestine operations. Lloyd Smith's original rescue mission in Albania was called "Champ."

The effort to finish the job in Albania was given a tellingly somber sobriquet: "Underdone." Until second lieutenants Ann Maness, Wilma Lytle, and Helen Porter could be sprung from Berat and spirited back to Italy, the combined job of OSS, SOE, and the resistance would not be done.

Extracting any Allied soldier from occupied Europe was daunting; trying to figure out how three Caucasian females could be slipped through a thicket of enemy troops in the middle of the Balkans was unprecedented. Underdone was "experiencing difficulty," the OSS Mediterranean desk reported to Bill Donovan's office in Washington in mid-January of 1944. Lloyd Smith asked for and received help: Four operational planners in Bari were assigned to his mission.

The Brits still inside Albania wanted the first crack at getting the three nurses out of Berat. Major Alan Palmer and Captain Victor Smith, who had been instrumental in refortifying the larger group in early December, had hoped to hike some forty miles northwest from Krushove, rendezvous with the nurses and their protectors somewhere in the mountains outside Berat, then escort them to Seaview.

Soon after Duffy and Lloyd Smith delivered the other twenty-seven Americans to Bari, Palmer and Victor Smith set out for Berat with a small party of LNC guides. But BK guerrillas ambushed them; Palmer and Smith were fortunate not to have been captured. They had no choice but to retreat to Krushove.

The SOE and the OSS developed a new plan, which once again involved bribing Balli strongmen, but this time procuring an automobile to handle the heavy portion of the journey. The plan hinged on persuading the three female officers to make and wear civilian clothes—an act that, if uncovered by the Germans, would have been punishable by death. Albanian guides would accompany them through hostile territory, keeping them in the car as long as the roads stayed safe. Once they ran out of passable highway, they would hike over the mountains.

At the other end, Lloyd Smith would again slip into Albania, bribe his way inland to Dukat through compliant BK leaders, meet up with Maness, Porter, and Lytle, and somehow get the trio over the last mountains and German lines to the Adriatic. It was another audacious plan; to pull it off, Smith and his team would need considerable on-the-ground help.

He got it after Hamilton's *Yankee* pulled into Gramma Bay, the location of Sea Elephant, the Allies' other coastal Albania intelligence base, around midnight on February 3. Smith's official report indicates that he met with SOE Major Anthony Quayle, the once

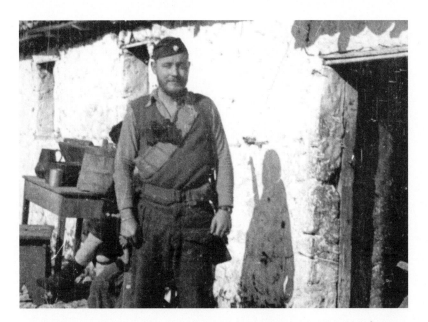

OSS Major Lloyd Smith behind Nazi lines in Albania, March 1944.

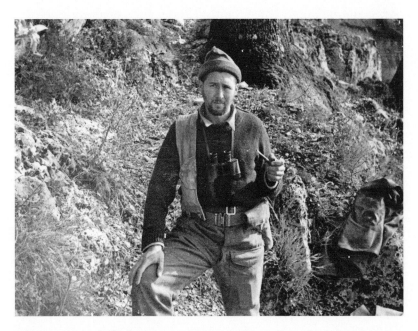

SOE Major and Shakespearean actor Anthony Quayle, February 1944.

and future thespian, at Sea Elephant, and an OSS major named "S. S. Kendall," who in truth was a civilian named Dale "Tank" McAdoo, a few miles farther north at Seaview. McAdoo was an upstate New Yorker who was heading OSS's skeletal mission in Albania.

Since Smith had again been armed in Bari with inducement gold, Kendall and Quayle, who got along handsomely for officers from rival agencies, suggested some well-placed coin would ensure the cooperation of local strongman (and OSS informant) Xheli Çela and his confrere, Hodo Meto, both of whom had powerful connections to the BK.

Given Tare Shyti's political and business savvy, there's an excellent chance he learned of the Americans' plight in late December or early January, when Smith was in negotiations with Xheli and Hodo. In all likelihood, Hodo, his first cousin, took Tare into his confidence when Smith explained the urgency of getting the three nurses out of Berat. Once Smith laid out the complexities of the rescue, Xheli and Hodo must have concluded that Tare was the best candidate to handle planning and execution.

The chieftains arranged for Tare to slip dressmaking material and forged documents to the nurses. Hodo also pledged to Smith that Tare would personally supervise the getaway.

There was little reason, Smith was then counseled by Kendall and Quayle, to head inland anytime soon. It would take weeks to make all the arrangements to get the nurses to Dukat; better for Smith to hang out at Seaview and Sea Elephant and line up his private army for the final push.

On February 12, local scouts reported that German patrols were getting perilously close to stumbling onto the Allies' coastal hideaways. The scouts believed it would be only a matter of days before the Germans launched an attack.

Smith conducted a reconnaissance of Seaview and discovered an encampment of enemy soldiers a few miles north at Orso Bay.

He posted sentinels disguised as shepherds to ensure that any German movement would be quickly detected.

The American officer, who'd just been promoted to major, was now worried about the three nurses arriving at the coastal bases only to find the outposts in enemy hands. He and his radio operator, Marine sergeant Nick R. Cooky, an Ohioan, agreed that if the Germans were to attack, they'd bury Cooky's radio battery for use another day and head for the hills.

Smith used Hodo's and Shyti's back channels to issue a warning to Midhat Fasheri, the titular head of Albania's collaborationist government, threatening reprisals should harm come to the remaining nurses. If there were any delay in getting the nurses to safety, Smith told Fasheri, he would have no choice but to tell the Allies that Balli Kombëtar had obstructed the rescue. The nurses' blood would be on BK's hands—with harsh retribution to follow.

The tough talk produced the desired results; Shyti, a skilled photographer, was given the resources he needed to wire counterfeit credentials in Tirana. With Major Smith's assent, the two cousins hatched a plot every bit as daring as the *Argo* rescue of American hostages in Teheran three and a half decades later.

Nosy German patrols coming from both the north and south were spotted along the coast on the morning of February 26. Seaview and Sea Elephant were immediately evacuated. Sergeant Cooky buried his extra radio battery and rendezvoused with Major Smith at a prearranged spot. With the enemy closing in, Quayle, the senior officer in charge, ordered the remaining SOE personnel to split into three groups and head east over the Dukati range.

Smith and Cooky hiked up a peak to its snowline—then hid in a gulley until dark. They slogged through four-foot-high snow; the wind was so vicious that, every few steps, it knocked them backward. Just shy of the summit, Smith and Cooky waited out the storm underneath a rock outcropping. They each grabbed a blanket from their backpack and shivered through the sleet. Smith was convinced he hadn't slept a wink, but Cooky assured him that in between teeth chatters, he snored. It took them hours the next morning to scale the summit and get below the snowline on the opposite side.

The next day, February 27, the pair spotted a six-man German patrol, which clearly saw them at the same time. But they eluded the enemy soldiers by pretending to head down the mountain; once they got out of the patrol's sight line and reached a wooded area, they doubled back up the hill without being followed.

Smith, Cooky, Quayle, and the others found safe quarters in Dukat and lay low, hoping to hear encouraging news from Hodo and Shyti. But another German offensive had disrupted Tare's route to Berat.

"If my cousin does not return within ten days," Hodo vowed to Smith on March 10, "you can shoot me. I'll bet my life on him."

On top of the German push, it turned out that the nurses' credentials had taken extra time to procure, despite Tare's photographic skills, Smith and Hodo's money, and Midhat's imprimatur.

On March 14, Smith received a radio message telling him that if the nurses could not be successfully evacuated within the next thirty days, he should return to Bari. The message rattled Hodo and the OSS-SOE brain trust in Albania; they were running out of options. They decided that if the nurses didn't get out by March 21, Smith would assemble as much firepower as he could and march to Berat to spring them.

Well into February, the Berat trio had still not dared leave the farmhouse. They took to heart the local leader's order to stay out of sight. Was the leader acting out of compassion? Or because

Hodo's network had paid him off? Or perhaps because he feared reprisals if the nurses were harmed? Whatever the reason, the Americans stayed safe.

The only time they left the property came one evening in early March, when the leader unexpectedly showed up with a car— quite likely the prospective getaway vehicle—and asked whether they wanted to go for a drive.

"It was nice just to get out," Maness remembered. "We went toward the hills and back. That is the only time we saw him [the leader]. No one else dared take us out, even though I think every-one in town knew we were there. Nobody bothered us."

Other than that liberating moment, they whiled away the hours playing cards with Mama. The Karajas' farmhouse was comfortable but had no running water or indoor plumbing. The water came from a deep well located beyond the outhouse in the backyard.

They were consigned to the farmhouse for a long ecclesiastical stretch: Advent, Christmas, and Lent. Since the Karajas were Orthodox, together they celebrated the holidays. Although meat was forbidden during Lent, the family served the Americans scraps of lamb and chicken, knowing they needed protein for their big undertaking. One day during Lent, Mama emerged from the kitchen rattling a pot with a big spoon, yelling, "Beans, beans, beans!"—the one word of English she'd mastered.

Her nephew, Nani's brother, knew a little English and often stopped in to reassure the nurses that the rescue operation was still on.

On March 15, exactly four months after the German attack on Berat, two English-speaking Albanians arrived at the farmhouse bearing dressmaking material. They briefed the women about the escape plan and urged them to begin making peasant frocks. With help from Goni and Mama, they fashioned dresses and large black scarves to cover their faces so they'd blend in. They would have only a few days to get ready, they were told.

"[The leaders] told us whatever we did, not to look the men in the eye. It would be a dead giveaway in two ways for Helen and Wilma, because they had blue eyes," Maness remembered.

On March 18, a man who refused to divulge his real name came to the house and told the nurses it was time to leave. It was Tare Shyti.

Wearing their peasant garb, they said fond farewells to their hosts, fastened their burqas, then slipped out a basement back door and climbed into the waiting sedan. As they pulled out onto the road, they were surprised that a truck full of Albanian soldiers began following them. The nurses didn't know it, but roughly half the soldiers in the truck were LNC Partisans, the other half BK guerrillas.

It was all part of Hodo and Tare's ruse: When stopped by German patrols or BK sentinels, Tare would produce a letter giving him permission to make the journey. The pretext was that the soldiers were being transported across the country to help the Germans fight the Partisans. It worked. Although sentries forced it to stop several times, the caravan worked its way west without being uncovered.

Maness, in the front passenger's seat, found herself literally riding shotgun. As they exited Berat, Tare, the driver, wordlessly handed her his rifle, which she kept at her feet.

"There was no way out, just hold the gun, look at the floor, and don't raise your eyes," she recalled.

Both the sedan and the truck had bad tires. A few hours into the journey, Tare was fixing a flat when a company of German soldiers stopped to investigate. They never gave the ladies a second look as they glanced at Tare's papers, tarrying for only a few moments before moving on.

During another stop at a BK checkpoint, armed guerrillas nosed around the car but never got suspicious.

They got as close to Dukat as they could—within a day's hike of Dukati Mountain—but ran out of decent road. The car and truck returned to Berat while the three Americans, Tare, and several of Shyti's handpicked guides walked along muddy trails.

They spent that night in a shepherd's hut. They were back up at dawn pushing toward Dukat. As twilight approached, they were thrilled to be greeted by two uniformed British soldiers waiting for them in a safe home.

Major Smith had spent that night in a hideaway cavern between Dukat and the coast. At 0700, he was shaken awake by an excitable English corporal. Smith, fearing the Germans were at that instant storming the cave, lunged for his service revolver.

But the corporal was trying to communicate good news. He finally managed to stammer, "The nurses have arrived!"

When Smith passed the news on to Hodo, the strongman exclaimed, "See, goddamn it, Major, I told you my cousin would bring them."

Smith's official report found the nurses in "the best possible physical condition" and said they were grateful to the actions of the BK—which was Smith's way of paying back Hodo and Xheli.

Having reached Dukat, the nurses still needed to get over the final mountain and down the coastal thoroughfare to Seaview, which once again was controlled by Allied intelligence since the Germans had evacuated the area.

On the night of March 19, Smith waited until sunset before transporting the nurses down the Valona-Dukat road. Once again, one of the rambling homes in the BK orbit was used to conceal and feed the Americans.

They spent most of the next day resting at Xheli's place along the coastal road. At eleven thirty that night, Smith led the three in a careful climb up the mountain. By dawn on the twenty-first they were high enough that any German patrol operating along the road would have been rendered impotent. Still, the ascent was scary and treacherous. Thick snow covered the top of the mountain.

They finally got to the summit just before noon and reached Seaview five hours later. To rest, Maness, Lytle, and Porter bunked in the same cots that their colleagues had used two and a half months earlier.

It wasn't until nearly midnight on March 21 that an Italian motorboat steered by an OSS pilot—but not Hamilton or his *Yankee* this time—sneaked away from the Albanian shore. It took thirteen rough hours to cross the strait. The nurses were "very seasick," Smith reported. They pulled into Otranto, Italy, at 1330 on March 22, 1944, without fanfare, an entourage, or popping flashbulbs.

Later that day, they enjoyed tea aboard a yacht that belonged to a Yugloslav friend of the OSS. On the morning of March 23, the nurses were taken by ambulance to the hospital in Bari, where all three were pronounced in remarkably good health.

The saga of "Underdone" was finally, mercifully, done. As Jens put it in her memoir, "The Albanian escape was now complete."

Whether it was the Balkan street smarts of Hasan Jina and Steffa Kostig, the sleight-of-hand of Tare Shyti, the tart tongue of Lois Watson McKenzie, the unblinking fealty of Garry Duffy, the well-placed cash of Lloyd Smith, the prayer book of Orville Abbott, the painstaking notes of Agnes Jensen, or the beans in Mama's pot, somehow thirty Americans survived all that time behind Nazi lines without suffering more than a scratch.

NEVER TOO LATE
TO SALUTE HEROES

There should have been a grand welcome-home reception at the White House, with newsreel cameras whirring, FDR reading a congratulatory message from Churchill, and Mrs. Roosevelt beaming as the nurses received their medals. Louisville should have thrown a ticker-tape parade, with Senator Happy Chandler and Major Red McKnight dedicating a building at Bowman Field in the 807th's honor.

Orville Abbott's memoir should have been a 1946 bestseller. Agnes Jensen should have serialized her story in *McCall's*. While back home in the Muskegon valley, the two Michiganders could have posed together for a pictorial spread in *Life*.

There should have been a 1947 Warner Brothers blockbuster called *Escape from Albania* directed by the great Michael Curtiz. He would have depicted the C-53's crash-landing in the same wonderfully cheesy way he shot the getaway plane zooming over the murky airdrome in *Casablanca*.

Studio head Jack Warner would have arranged for Barbara Stanwyck to play Agnes Jensen. Cary Grant would have played Lieutenant Garry Duffy, of course, complete with an over-the-top Yorkshire accent. Anthony Quinn would have played Hasan, his handlebar mustache stretching from one ear to the other. Quinn would have used Hasan's verbal tic "Never mind!" to great comedic effect. Claude Rains, a Curtiz favorite, would have mastered a Balkan accent and portrayed the oily Steffa to perfection.

Hollywood would have changed the story to include a furtive romance between Jens and Duffy. The movie would have ended with violins surging as Stanwyk and Grant share a final salty kiss in Bari, with Garry/Cary vowing to return to harm's way to serve the cause of freedom and Jens/Babs purring that she'll never forget him.

There should have been a twentieth-anniversary gathering in Berat, where the erstwhile castaways would have been reunited with Duffy, Blondie, Lloyd Smith, Victor Smith, Hasan, Steffa, Tare, Johnny, and their other Albanian rescuers. The cameras of *CBS Reports* would have been there to capture the moment in the Kolumbos' dining room when they toasted their mutual valor in thwarting Hitler's Reich.

All this should have happened, but sadly, none of it did. The Albanian odyssey of the 807th Medical Air Evacuation Squadron ended up falling through the cracks of history. Not only was there no medal ceremony—there were no special military commendations at all. There was next to no official acknowledgment of their ordeal; nor was there any compensation for the hardship they had endured. Military nurses who had survived the nightmare of Bataan and Corregidor were given White House receptions and warm public recognition—but not the nurses who survived the nightmare of Albania.

The only "medal" Orville Abbott received was facetious. While serving stateside in the spring of 1944 with the 805th MAES at the Army Air Forces' Tactical Center in Orlando, Abbott and Bob Owen were inducted into the "U.S. Late Arrival Club." It was a special fraternity of MTO soldiers who managed to "walk back" to friendly lines after being trapped in enemy territory. The July 14, 1944, edition of *Yank*, the Army's weekly magazine, ran a photo and a blurb mentioning that Owen and Abbott were each "presented with an emblem, which is in the shape of a boot with wings." Most of the others in the 807th didn't even get that token recognition.

Not unlike Jens's responsibility at Bowman Field, Orville's job with the 805th that spring was to fly to ports of embarkation around the country, showing medic trainees how to treat wounded soldiers. In the fall of 1944, he was transferred to the AAF 501st in Palm Springs, California, and a few months later to the 349th at Baer Airfield in Indiana.

At some point in 1944, unbeknownst to Owen and his other 807th pals, Abbott began taking his Albanian diary notes (which apparently he had kept concealed during G-2 questioning in Bari) and distilling them into book form. While home in Michigan on leave, he shared his handwritten notes with reporter and editor Allen Field Smith of the *Newaygo Republican*. They shook hands on a partnership; by late summer of 1945— after many a late night hammering away at Smith's typewriter— they had produced a 242-page manuscript called *Albanian Episode*.

Abbott and Smith defanged the story so it protected the identity of Albanian Partisans and Allied special ops soldiers and obscured the 807th's escape route. After submitting it for review in September of 1945, they ended up getting a surprisingly quick green light from military censors. Soon they hired a New York–based literary agent named Ann Elmo. She shopped the book around, but remarkably, no publisher bit.

Abbott, discouraged, didn't bother to keep a copy of the manuscript. Six years later, when Orville wed his wife, Verda, he never mentioned that he'd written a book, and kept his silence through three decades of marriage. Verda only had the vaguest sense of what her husband had gone through in Albania.

In the early 1950s, Abbott joined the United Auto Workers and got a job at the Fisher Body metal stamping plant in Grand Rapids. He stayed at the Fisher facility for thirty years. In 1960, Abbott indulged his lifelong interest in politics by running for a state assembly seat as a Democrat. Had he played up his wartime heroics he might have won. But he didn't; he had too much dignity. He lost.

As the years went by, his writing partner also forgot about *Albanian Episode*. Allen Smith stuck the manuscript in a cardboard box, where it collected dust.

Abbott almost never talked about the war in front of son Clint or daughters Holly and Lori, dismissing his experience with a shrug of the shoulders. "Don't live in the past," he would advise the inquisitive Clint, who as a kid liked to sneak up to the attic and open his dad's AAF footlocker.

About a year before Lawrence Orville Abbott died in 1982 of complications from heart bypass surgery, he opened up about Albania—at least a little—one night while the family was sitting around the kitchen table sipping Cokes. Sometimes all the American castaways had to sleep in the same room, he said to his wife's and kids' amazement. He also told his family how indebted he was to the Albanians who'd helped them, how he'd always felt guilty that he hadn't thanked them.

Nineteen years after his dad's death, Clint bumped into his uncle George one morning at the Newaygo post office. George had been hectoring Clint to write an article for the local paper about his dad's escapade.

"You know, he wrote a book about this," George volunteered.

Clint was stunned. "He did? I don't think we have it, but I'll look," he told his uncle.

Clint pulled out his dad's footlocker and found a lot of fascinating mementos but no manuscript. But it was now the age of the Internet; a yellowing *Grand Rapids Press* story from February 24, 1944, led Clint to Agnes Jensen Mangerich, who in turn encouraged Clint to get in touch with Elna Schwant, Jim Cruise, Harold Hayes, and other surviving members of the 807th. Clint's research intensified.

Eventually Uncle George remembered the name of his brother's old writing partner. Through the Newaygo High alumni association, Clint discovered Allen Smith's daughter Marcia Smith Claus living in Houston. As they talked on the phone, Marcia remembered coming home from school as a teenager and seeing her dad and Clint's dad working hard around a typewriter. She said she still had some of her father's old boxes and would wade through them.

Many months later Marcia called to say that she'd found the manuscript, completely intact, along with original handwritten notes from Clint's dad.

Clint revamped his dad's book, incorporating facts, individual identities, and village names from meager press accounts and from Agnes Jensen Mangerich's memoir, which by then had been out for several years. What emerged was *Out of Albania—From the Memoirs of Lawrence O. Abbott: A True Account of a World War II Underground Rescue Mission*. Clint self-published it in 2010.

Jens stayed in the AAF nursing corps until a year after V-E Day, earning three decorations, including a World War II Victory Medal. In the immediate postwar years, Jens had no idea that Abbott had attempted to publish his own book and, in fact, had obtained authorization from military authorities. She wanted to convert her diary notes into something publishable, but felt obliged to wait until Enver Hoxha's Communist regime had completely collapsed, lest the dictator seek revenge against countrymen who—at least in his fetid little mind—had remained loyal to the West after they helped the Americans escape.

Jens had a long wait. *Vdekje Fashizmit* proved a triumph, *Liri Popullit* a cruel joke. As 1944 wore on and the Third Reich began hemorrhaging from all sides, Hitler and von Weichs became even more despicable in their treatment of the Balkans. Lytle, Maness, and Porter were in the midst of sewing their escape garb when the Wehrmacht launched another assault against central and southern Albania. SOE's own analysis acknowledges that the Germans overran the LNC's "centres of resistance" south of Valona, in Gjirokastër, and at Korçë, slaughtering hundreds of innocents.

But the enemy atrocities served to swell the ranks of Hoxha's LNC. At a conference in Përmet two months after the last three nurses had escaped, Hoxha was officially named supreme commander of Albania's national liberation army. With sustained support from SOE, the Albanian *komitadjis* became a formidable force. By mid-1944, the SOE had parachuted in some fifteen thousand rifles, Sten guns, and machine guns, plus twenty-five thousand grenades, to Hoxha's army. Buttressed by this new firepower, the LNC was able to take the offensive against the Nazi occupiers and their collaborators.

In June 1944, as the Allies established a beachhead in northern France, pressure from the Partisans forced the Reich to move its crack 1st Mountain Division from the Russian front to Albania in a futile bid to exterminate the LNC in southern Albania. "The

Partisans melted away before them," the SOE reported, "but once again lost no time in re-forming as the tide receded."

Within weeks the LNC had effectively counterattacked. Hoxha's SOE-trained and -equipped division of more than ten thousand soldiers, male and female, drove north of the 807th's crash site along the Shkumbini. For the next month, the SOE noted, "a bloodthirsty battle raged." The Germans had no choice but to begin their retreat from Greece, Albania, and Yugoslavia sooner than they had planned, especially when the RAF intensified its strafing of Wehrmacht encampments, and British commandos pulled off a series of daring behind-the-lines raids.

Surely Hasan and Pandee—maybe even Johnny—fought in the great LNC offensive. The Germans so feared annihilation that they demolished every bridge and road in their wake.

On November 5, the Germans and their Balli mercenaries abandoned Elbasan, Hasan's home territory, and began a fierce retreat north. The BK "fell to pieces," SOE asserted. Hoxha soon headed a triumphal parade through the streets of Tirana. On the final day of November 1944, "the last German column quitted Albanian soil," wrote SOE.

A confidential SOE report suggests that in the fifteen months between late summer 1943 and the German withdrawal in the fall of 1944, Albanian Partisans had accounted for "7-8,000 Germans killed, 500 captured, and 600 MT [motor transport] vehicles destroyed or captured." It was, the special ops agency concluded, an achievement of overriding strategic significance; it forced the Germans to withdraw troops from the Russian front while preventing others from joining the Wehrmacht's defense of France after D-Day.

Alas, the persecution of the Albanian people did not end with the Nazi retreat. Once he consolidated power, Hoxha snuffed out all opposition, real or imagined. Unlike Tito, Hoxha became a Russian sycophant behind what Churchill would soon brand the Iron Curtain. Hoxha was such a dedicated ideologue that he broke away from the Soviet Union during Nikita Khrushchev's anti-Stalin takeover in the mid- to late 1950s, ultimately aligning himself with Chairman Mao's China, which Hoxha viewed as the true inheritor of the Lenin-Stalin legacy. Albania under Hoxha stayed as oppressive and insular as it had under outside conquerors. Even worse, Hoxha forged a cult of megalomania akin to Kim Jong Il's in North Korea.

Hoxha punished thousands of Albanians for such innocuous "crimes" as being found with an English dictionary or reading a magazine that could be construed as capitalist or pro-Western. Among his victims, sadly, were Kostig Steffa, Xheli Çela, and Tare Shyti.

Soon after the war ended, Steffa was arrested and jailed near Berat, apparently for being insufficiently loyal to the state. In 1947, the cosmopolitan school superintendent and father of five, the man who had spent seven harrowing weeks guiding desperate Americans through Fascist territory, was executed by a Communist firing squad.

Xheli was abandoned by Allied intelligence after the war and had no choice but to flee to Italy. Hoxha's hit men tracked him down and murdered him.

Given Hoxha's zealotry against anyone allied with the Balli Kompëtar, it's miraculous that Tare escaped Steffa's fate. Tare may not have been a BK member or even a Balli sympathizer, but he was a blood relative and close associate of Hodo Meto, like Xheli, one of Hoxha's despised adversaries. And Tare clearly subscribed to views that were pro-Western and prodemocracy. Toward the end of the war, Tare contemplated seeking asylum; he jumped over the back wall of the British embassy in Tirana. For whatever reason, however, Tare chose to reenter Albanian society, despite the risks.

Tare spent much of his life under house arrest, denied the right to work or travel. He and his wife had two more children, and eventually eleven grandchildren and seventeen great-grandchildren. The most recent Shyti great-grandchild was born in Tirana in the fall of 2012.

Shyti was no doubt determined to outlive Hoxha and see the dawn of a new era for his beloved Albania—but he fell short. Shyti died in 1983, two years before Hoxha succumbed to diabetes. Leka Bezhani, one of Tare's grandsons, and his mother, Tare's daughter, the seventy-seven-year-old Vojsava Shyti Bezhani, now live in Worcester, Massachusetts. Leka has served in both the Albanian army reserve and the Massachusetts National Guard, dual accomplishments that would have pleased his grandfather no end.

Hoxha, the avatar of the people's uprising, had managed over four decades to pile up a fortune that made King Zog look like a piker. A few years after Hoxha's death, when Communism collapsed throughout Eastern Europe, Albanians took delight in tearing down the statues and monuments that Hoxha had erected to himself, including his gravestone.

Today Albania is a capitalist democracy, albeit one struggling to catch up to the rest of Europe. The corrupt business practices and Ponzi schemes that have plagued the former Soviet bloc have been particularly crippling in Albania. Thousands have been bilked; joblessness remains endemic. But those problems pale in comparison to the ravages visited upon Shquiperi by *Liri Populitt* and before that, *Fashizmit.* Someday soon, Albania deserves to soar like an eagle.

The five-plus weeks it took for Hal Boyle's AP story—the *Hartford Courant* headlined it "American Nurses and Airmen

Saved After Thrilling Balkan Adventure"—to clear censors betrayed the wariness of U.S. military officials toward giving the 807th's exploits too much public exposure.

Already apprehensive about Stalin's postwar ambitions, American officials were more skittish about crediting pro-Soviet Partisans than their British counterparts, Jon Naar recalls. There may also have been nervousness that press scrutiny would inevitably invite questions about pilot error and the slipshod preparation that contributed to the 807th's flight getting so badly off course. Finally, the Americans were not keen about acknowledging the dominant role the Brits had played in rescuing the marooned Yanks.

After Germany's surrender, the episode got caught up in Cold War recrimination. This saga of Allied and resistance fortitude against unspeakable evil fell victim to superpower jockeying between East and West.

U.S. press coverage of the incident in the winter and spring of 1944 was sporadic and superficial. Besides the Boyle piece, there was little national play beyond brief mentions in *Stars and Stripes*. A few local papers—the *Detroit Free Press*, the *Grand Rapids Press*, and the *Big Rapids Pioneer*—ran short profiles of the 807th's returning heroines and heroes.

Life and *Look*, the weekly pictorials, never picked up the story. The best periodical treatment was in the April 1, 1944, *Collier's Weekly*, whose article centered on the two Detroit-area nurses, lieutenants Rutkowski and Tacina. Reporter Amy Porter's piece, entitled "Balkan Escape," ran roughly six thousand words and included a reasonable facsimile of some of the episode's cliffhanger moments, although there was no mention of Jean collapsing on Mount Tomorrit or Tassy tumbling down the mountain near Golem with Garry Duffy clinging to her belt. During the war, *Collier's* circulation topped two million, so it was not insignificant exposure.

Still, it was a comic-book depiction that probably left the biggest impression on the American populace. Two and a half years after V-E Day, the October 1947 *True Comics* ran a four-page, seventeen-panel strip also dubbed "Balkan Escape."

True (its marvelous tagline was "TRUTH is stranger and a thousand times more thrilling than FICTION!") messed up the episode's chronology, gave short shrift to the role of the Brits and Partisans, and portrayed the nurses as ersatz "Brenda Starrs," complete with pouty lips and décolletage. The pilots, naturally, were pictured as grizzled, take-charge types, coolly calling the shots on the attempted air rescue and the push to the coast.

Yet despite the constraints of space, *True* managed to distill the pathos of the Balkan ordeal into a single panel. In midstrip, the group is shown sitting on the stone floor of a crude hut, eating out of a pot.

The panel was headed: "Despite extreme poverty, the Albanians share their meager food supplies."

One of the nurses, a blonde, frets, "These people are starving."

A brunette responds, "I know. But we can't refuse to eat. They'd feel insulted. Let's leave some of our clothing for them."

At least comic-book readers learned of the astonishing generosity of the Albanian people.

The 1944 book *Mediterranean Sweep: Air Stories from El Alamein to Rome*, written by a pair of active-duty military officers, also presents a pilot-centric view of the odyssey. It's clear that Thrasher and Baggs were the principal sources for Major Richard Thruelsen, a prospective *Saturday Evening Post* editor, and Lieutenant Elliott Arnold, a once and future features writer for the *New York World-Telegram*.

In a twelve-page chapter entitled "Balkan Journey," the pair barely mentioned the Brits, and described the pilots as selflessly refusing to head for the hills during the enemy siege of Berat until all the nurses were accounted for. The truth, as Jens and Abbott documented, was far less flattering. Jean Rutkowski's daughter Lee remembers her mother expressing disdain toward Thrasher's decision making. The AAF's inquiry into the errant flight stopped short of a court-martial but reprimanded the crew for not following proper procedures.

Most of the Brits who valiantly guided the Americans to safety stayed in the Balkan sphere until the Nazis were ejected. Major Philip Leake, Jon Naar's boss and the SOE officer who vehemently deplored FDR's meddling, skulked into Albania against Naar's advice in 1944. Leake was killed in a Luftwaffe raid. Major C. Alan Palmer survived all those months behind Nazi lines and returned to English society and his family's biscuit fortune. Captain Victor Smith, who saved the party from being trapped by Ballis in the Albanian Alps, was awarded a Military Cross.

Sergeant H. J. "Blondie" Bell moved to Australia after the war, then returned to England and reveled in watching his grandchildren play soccer. Corporal Willie Williamson, one of the SOE's Albanian trailblazers, was dropped into northern Italy in mid-1944 and promptly captured. He spent the remainder of the war in a German stalag. Trained as a chemist, Williamson returned to his native Scotland, became a schoolteacher, and retired outside Edinburgh.

Major H. W. "Bill" Tilman, too, parachuted into Italy in 1944, avoided capture, and was ultimately awarded the Distinguished Service Order. After the war, the mountaineer shifted his energies to sailing and became a bestselling high-seas adventure writer. In 1977, Tilman set out in a sailboat from Rio de Janeiro, intent on reaching Britain's Falkland Islands off the Argentine coast. He was never heard from again.

Captain Jon Naar devoted two years of his life to helping liberate Albania. But the only time he set foot in the country was a cold night in early 1944, when his pal, U.S. Marine lieutenant John Hamilton, making a supply run, whisked him to Seaview and back aboard the *Yankee*.

After the Nazis were chased out of the Balkans, Naar was promoted to major and appointed head of counterintelligence planning for Austria at Allied Forces Headquarters in Caserta, Italy. Naar had some thirty intelligence operatives under his command, half of them American. The plan was to infiltrate his group into Vienna in early 1945—a mission rendered moot when the Red Army beat Patton's Third Army to the punch and rolled into the Austrian capital. The Naar group's new charge was to apprehend war criminals for prosecution at Nuremberg, a difficult task made more daunting, Naar says, by U.S. intelligence's recruiting of ex-Nazis to blunt the burgeoning influence of the Soviets.

One of the female OSS officers in Caserta was Captain Ellen Hartt, a Bostonian whom Naar courted and married. He came to the U.S. in the summer of 1946 as a "G.I. bridegroom," as he put it, and never left—despite an eventual divorce from Hartt. After serving as managing editor of Worldwide Medical News Service in New York, he became an acclaimed photographer, working for the *New York Times Magazine* and many other publications and clients. He has written or cowritten twelve books, ranging in subject from photography to solar energy to ecological sustainability.

Today, at ninety-three, he still looks spry enough to persuade Vichy Frenchmen, *en français*, to abandon the Reich and join the Allies, as he did for MI6 in Syria and Lebanon seven decades ago. In the winter and spring of 2013, sixty-two of Naar's signature photographs were featured in a highly praised exhibition at the New Jersey State Museum in Trenton.

SOE's Major David Smiley never lost his infatuation for Albania. Four years after the war ended, he helped engineer an ill-fated MI6 coup attempt to overthrow the Hoxha regime. The plan called for a special operations force recruited and led by Smiley to land on Albania's coast, then meet up with anti-Hoxha elements to upend the Communists.

Smiley's raid unraveled thanks to the Brits' misapprehension of Hoxha's strength, poor security, and a diabolical double cross executed by the first secretary to the British ambassador in Washington, D.C. The Cambridge University–trained turncoat was named Harold A. R. "Kim" Philby. Undetected by the Brits, Philby had been feeding secret information to the Soviets for close to two decades while at various British diplomatic and "journalistic" posts. He had gotten wind of the Albanian scheme and warned Moscow and Tirana. Hoxha's army, waiting in the weeds, shredded Smiley's forces in a debacle that presaged the failed Bay of Pigs operation in Cuba twelve years later.

The great soldier was fortunate to survive. He was eventually awarded an Order of the British Empire medal to go with his two Military Crosses. After completing his military career serving in various capacities in the Persian Gulf, he lived out his years on a farm in Spain.

Lieutenant Gavan Bernard "Garry" Duffy was never officially acknowledged by the U.S. military, an omission that caused a fair degree of bitterness in SOE circles.

"I must say that when I saw Duffy I thought he deserved the rank of Captain, and his very skillful and patient handling of the very difficult problem of evacuating the nurses seemed to me also to warrant some form of recognition," Major Leake wrote to an SOE colleague on May 30, 1944. "I thought at the time that perhaps some decoration might have been awarded him by the Americans as a gesture of courtesy, but one has heard nothing of it so far."

America's silence deepened as the months and years went by. Duffy was indeed awarded a promotion to captain as he was assigned to SOE headquarters in Bari. Since he'd had only two short leaves in five-plus years of wartime service, he was given an extended sabbatical in the spring of 1944 to visit his family in Leeds. Duffy took ill in transit and was hospitalized. He recovered and became an SOE demolitions trainer in the U.K. Before war's end, he was again committed to active duty in the Mediterranean.

In peacetime, Duffy stayed in His Majesty's army as a recruiter. He eventually got his wish and returned to the north, assigned to Wirral, Merseyside, not far from his boyhood home. He married a woman named Dyllis, with whom he shared virtually nothing of his cloak-and-dagger years in the Balkans. They never had children.

Even after retiring from the army in 1961, Major Duffy stayed in Wirral. An avid golfer, he joined Royal Liverpool, the fabled Hoylake links hard by the Irish Sea. He no doubt was in the gallery, or more likely serving as a marshal, when Argentinian Roberto De Vicenzo beat American Jack Nicklaus in a memorable Open Championship at Royal Liverpool in 1967. He stayed an active member until he passed away in 1990, at the age of seventy.

Agnes Jensen happened to bump into C. B. Thrasher at a stateside air base a couple of months after V-E day. Jens asked whether Thrasher knew what had become of Duffy. The pilot told her that he'd heard Duffy had been killed while parachuting into Germany on a secret mission.

When Jens found out five decades later that Duffy had for forty-five years been very much alive and living in England, she regretted taking Thrasher at his word. She would love to have

visited with Duffy and to have invited him to attend one of the
807th's reunions.

After the war, the escapees came home, tried to lead "normal" lives, found work and marriage, started families, and became
part of the wondrous generation that built postwar America. Like
so many World War II veterans, most rarely talked about their
searing experiences. Agnes Jensen Mangerich's two children,
Karen and Jon, didn't know the extent of the 807th's story until
they became adults. The same essentially held true for Larry
Abbott's children, Lois Watson McKenzie's kids, and Gayle Lebo,
Dick's daughter.

The exception was Jean Rutkowski's daughter, Lee, who while
growing up heard tons of stories from her voluble mother. Jean had
come home to the Detroit area after the war and gotten a job at
the local Veterans Administration hospital. She fell in love with a
wounded vet whom she was treating and married him. Jean
enjoyed recounting stories about her two-month trek through
Albania, most of them lighthearted, with Lee and her grandchildren. After Jean's husband passed away, she moved to Phoenix to
live with Lee's family. Jean died in 2009.

For the most part, the Albanian castaways lost touch.
Phyllis McKenzie remembers her mother, Lois, lamenting that she
didn't have her 807th friends' addresses when she sent out Christmas cards.

Harold Hayes did have Larry Abbott's address, at least for a
time. In January 1961, Harold wrote his "Bro Abbott" a belated
Christmas letter that matter-of-factly described what his kids were

up to and his latest challenges on the factory floor as an aeronauti-cal executive—without even hinting at the trauma they'd shared two decades before.

In 1983, a year after Abbott's passing, with the fortieth anni-versary of the crash-landing looming, Hayes, still living on the West Coast, organized the first official reunion of the 807th. Har-old's brother Karl offered his home in Columbus, Ohio, for the occa-sion. On the first night, an Associated Press reporter witnessed the sixty-one-year-old Gilbert Hornsby, still residing in his native Manchester, Kentucky, greet the sixty-six-year-old Gertrude Daw-son Hill, then of Charles Town, West Virginia.

"Of course I remember you," Tooie told Gilbert. "You saved my life."

Of all the stories they shared, it was their reminiscences about scaling icy summits like Mount Tomorrit, where Hornsby stopped Dawson from sliding to near-certain death, that made the biggest impression on the reporter. Hayes was quoted as saying, "There was a lot of frustration. We'd climb up a mountain and get to the top, and then we'd see another mountain ahead we'd have to climb."

Jens, then living in Bethesda, Maryland, was among those who brought along a scrapbook. They had a grand time poring over maps, trying to figure out how they'd gotten from place to place. Among the attendees were Jim Cruise of Brockton, Massachu-setts; Charlie Adams of Edwardsburg, Michigan; Bob Owen of Gulfport, Mississippi; Lois Watson McKenzie of Topeka, Kansas; and Elna Schwant Krumm of Allegan, Michigan.

Right after the war, Jens married Harry Leo Mangerich, a tax auditor with the U.S. Agency for International Development. The Mangerichs lived all over, including Japan, Taiwan, Guam, Afghanistan, Nicaragua, and northern California, before settling outside Washington, D.C. Jens and Lieutenant Colonel Lloyd G. Smith renewed their acquaintance when the Mangerichs lived in Maryland and Smith, then finishing up a distinguished military intelligence career in Washington, was living in a lovely country home in Vienna, Virginia. The two got together often in the eighties and the nineties. Jens persuaded Lloyd to attend an 807th reunion, where he jotted down his memories and was applauded as one of their redeemers. Smith passed away in 2005.

Jens enjoyed going to the medical flight evacuation reunions and gatherings of the Air Forces Escape and Evasion Society. Out of the blue in 1995, a reporter from the *Liverpool* (U.K.) *Daily Post* named Harold Brough telephoned Jens. Brough was calling at the prodding of a former golfing buddy of Garry Duffy's named John Graham. Graham had served in postwar British intelligence and was fascinated by his late friend's World War II exploits in the Balkans.

Duffy had died five years earlier, Brough told Jens. But with Dyllis Duffy's help, Graham and Brough had unearthed some of the old demolitionist's reports on the Albanian rescue.

Jens, then eighty, immediately expressed regret that she hadn't known Duffy had been alive for all those years. "I don't know why I was so dumb as to believe he had been killed," she told Brough. Her own husband, Harry, had passed away three years earlier. As far as Jens knew at that point, only four other 807th nurses were still alive. She told Brough:

> I remember we girls could not resist teasing him [Duffy]. He used to look at us, perhaps thinking one might have a hysterical fit. I remember him one night watching this girl putting her hair up and saying he did not even have sisters. Meaning here he was surrounded by all these women!
>
> He was never nasty or mean. He was standoffish, but that was necessary to maintain discipline. We never questioned him, because he was in control. He was a leader.

I used to think what might happen if someone got sick or broke a leg or something. That was always on my mind. It would have been disastrous. I do not think I ever realized just what was involved in keeping us clear of the other side. But I always believed he would get us out.

The *Daily Post* piece quoted from one of Duffy's after-action reports: "[The nurses] always managed to create an impression either leaving or entering a village . . . they always managed to produce the necessary cosmetics and render the necessary running repairs. They left the people nonplussed, including myself. After all, they were in enemy-occupied territory. Amazing."

Amazing indeed. As Jens told Brough: "We owe him our lives."

That same year, 1995, Jens went to Albania with her two children on a trip organized by Boston journalist and Albanian historian Peter Lucas. They visited Dukat and sat in the home of onetime Xheli Çela acolyte Isuf Shehaj. It was the place where, fifty-two years earlier, Jens and her friends had been revived with hot tea on their push to the coast.

With the help of Çestie's village elders, they found the crash site and learned that for many years afterward, people in the surrounding area would help themselves to pieces of the C-53's wreckage, proudly displaying the shards in their homes. By the time Jens and her family visited, though, the debris had been picked clean. There was nothing left in the old lakebed to suggest it was where a mustachioed guerrilla leader had come galloping to the rescue on a white horse.

In Berat, Jens visited with Kostig Steffa's widow and heard firsthand the story of Hoxha's hideous revenge five decades before.

Sadly, Steffa's son Alfredo, the boy to whom Jens had given her aviator's wings in January of 1944, had been suffering from a long-term illness and died the day after Jens spoke with his mother. The Albanian government gave Jens a much-belated medal for bravery.

Jean Rutkowski, her daughter now says, felt so indebted to Steffa's family that for years she sent money to his widow. Surely other members of the 807th were equally generous.

Lucas brought back to Brockton, Massachusetts, a piece of the C-53 for the larger-than-life old medic Jim Cruise. Cruise loved showing it off to friends, of whom he had many. For thirty-three years, Jim served as supervisor of letter carriers in Brockton's post office. His signature greeting was, "Gawd love ya." When in the early 2000s Clint Abbott informed Cruise that his father, Larry, had passed away two decades before, Cruise exclaimed, "Larry Abbott! Gawd love him! If Larry Abbott isn't in heaven, then what in the hell chance does a guy like myself have?" The man who bellowed at Agnes Jensen to pull down his hat in the middle of Mount Tomorrit's blizzard died in 2010, leaving nine grandchildren.

As he began in earnest to research his dad's story, Clint reached out to Jens and other 807th survivors. In August 2001, two years after the publication of Jens's memoir, *Albanian Escape*, Clint hosted Jens and Elna Schwant Krumm in Newaygo. Thirty western Michiganders and a reporter/photographer with the *Newaygo County Times* gathered at the River Stop Café to listen to the C-53 seatmates recount their memories. The two octogenerians may have been a little hunched over and gray—but they didn't miss a beat.

Elna revealed that early on in Albania, she quietly asked a male colleague what they were eating. "Never mind, eat it!" he hissed back.

"The people were so desperately poor," Elna told the crowd.

"They risked their lives in opening their houses to us," Jens affirmed.

Elna and Jens also shared this sprightly anecdote: While in the Brits' care in Krushove, the nurses had been promised a shipment of new undergarments. Sadly, the women's underwear was dumped via parachute a day *after* they bugged out. The delivery chute apparently missed its mark: They heard scuttlebutt that the lingerie ended up in enemy hands.

"We always wanted to see the Germans' faces when they found that box. They must have wondered what [the Brits] needed that for," Jens said, to the crowd's amusement.

Elna's brother, Navy lieutenant (jg) Willard Henry Schwant, was officially declared killed in action before the war ended. He had gone missing on August 3, 1943, thirteen weeks before his sister's plane crashed inside the Reich. Winner, South Dakota, their hometown, had fewer than twenty-five hundred inhabitants. With two of the Schwant kids missing, and the other two away on active duty, there could not have been much joy in Winner during the 1943 Christmas holidays.

Willard Henry's sister died in 2008, two years before her pal Jens. The responsive reading at Jens's memorial service in La Jolla, California, began with an excerpt from Romans 8:35.

> Who shall separate us from the love of Christ? Shall tribulation, or distress, or persecution, or famine, or nakedness, or peril, or sword?

In her sixty-two days in Albania and in her ninety-five years on earth, Agnes Anna Jensen Mangerich surmounted almost all of those biblical plagues. Garry Duffy wasn't the only person she left nonplussed.

Not all the refugees' lives turned out as long or as fulfilled as Jens's, but, on balance, they did pretty well. The three nurses who took scary tumbles in the Albanian snow—Gertrude "Tooie" Dawson Tiedeken, Lillian "Tassy" Tacina Ratag, and Eugenie Helen Rutkowski Wilkinson—all got married, had families, and lived at least into their seventies.

Two of the feisty Berat seamstresses—Ava Ann Maness and Wilma Lytle—led long lives devoted to nursing. Ann made it to eighty-two; Wilma to ninety-three. Helen Porter died young, at fifty-six.

The first member of the troupe to pass away was Jens's bunkmate the morning the Germans attacked Berat: Ann Kopsco. She died in 1967, at age fifty-five. Paula Kanable was killed in an automobile accident at sixty-six in 1983. Chicagoan Ann Markowitz died in 2005. Among the men, Jim Baggs, the coon-hunting co-pilot, was the first to go, dying in 1978 at age sixty-two. Paul Allen, the slap-happy teenager, lived until 1982. Thrasher, the ill-starred pilot, passed away in 1990. Shumway, the crew chief with the bum knee, died in 2000.

Dick Lebo, the radioman, spent the better part of four decades as the postmaster of Halifax, Pennsylvania. His daughter, Gayle Lebo Yost, was awestruck while reading Jens's book; until then, she had little appreciation for the anguish her dad had experienced. Around 2008, with Dick still alive, Gayle wrote a letter to the local newspaper, the *Harrisburg Patriot-News*, suggesting a Memorial Day feature on her father's World War II service. But when the reporter called, her dad demurred.

"I know you spent a lot of time writing that letter and I hope you understand," he told Gayle. "There were a lot of people who did what I did."

He imbued a sense of patriotic duty in his children and grand-children. One of the proudest days of his life was when his grand-son, Gayle's nephew, received a Silver Star for heroism in Iraq.

Dick Lebo died in 2010. His funeral service ended with the playing of the Air Force hymn. Sixty-seven years earlier, off he'd gone into the wildest blue yonder any airman could imagine.

Prewar life had not been easy for Lois Eileen Watson in the rough-and-tumble South Side. Postwar life, too, proved diffi-cult. After serving as a nurse at stateside military hospitals, she reunited with Nolan. Her husband had flown a thousand hours as a B-24 flight commander assigned, coincidentally, to the 15th U.S. Army Air Force. His squadron attacked targets in Germany, Aus-tria, and northern Italy.

Lois confided in the husband whom she barely knew that her Albanian experience had changed her. She was less effusive about life, more jaded. If Nolan wanted out of the marriage, she would understand. Her least favorite photo was a shot taken with her hus-band a few months after the war. It made her eyes look so sad, she would tell her daughter Phyllis.

The couple moved to Manhattan, Kansas, so Nolan could get his master's in business administration at Kansas State. Lois served as house mother of Nolan's old fraternity, Pi Kappa Alpha. Nolan then accepted a position with the Commerce Acceptance Com-pany, first in Kansas City for three years, then in Topeka, which they made their permanent home. Their third child, a boy follow-ing two girls, came along in 1952.

Two years later, Lois got a job as a nurse at the Topeka Veterans Administration hospital, working with World War II, Korean War, and, in the sixties, seventies, and eighties, Vietnam-era combat veterans suffering from what was then called shell shock. Today the condition is known as post-traumatic stress disorder; its disquieting symptoms include depression, social anxiety, and substance abuse.

While working all those years with scarred veterans, Lois must have suffered from her own form of PTSD. She struggled with melancholia and alcohol dependence, especially after her second child, Paula Jean, was killed in a tragic 1975 car accident on a New Mexico mountain. Spirited and vivacious, Paula had just graduated from Kansas University Medical School and was serving that summer as a physician at the Philmont Boy Scout camp. As a young doctor, she was leading the independent life that, in many ways, Lois herself had wanted to live. Paula was twenty-four, essentially the same age her mother had been when she was trapped in Albania. Lois had managed to survive one hilltop mishap after another while being chased by Nazis and Barleys. It must have been unfathomable that her daughter could be killed on a mountainside while doing something as carefree as working at a camp.

Paula's death devastated Lois and Nolan. It could not have helped that Lois was surrounded every day at the hospital with people beset by their own demons.

Her drinking became so heavy that twice she checked herself into rehabilitation programs. In both instances she was able to stop for a while but suffered relapses. Lois's fondest wish, Phyllis says, was that the 807th's saga be better known and appreciated. She took a gold sovereign that the Brits had given her as a souvenir and turned it into a pendant; for years she wore it around her neck. Still, she never wrote down her Albanian recollections until 1983, when a substance abuse counselor asked her to do it as part of her therapy.

Lois produced a cathartic little autobiography full of touching insights. She used her memoir to shape a 1991 presentation she made as a panelist at a forum on wartime nursing at Topeka's Washburn University. Lois enjoyed the Washburn program; her picture and story were highlighted in the *Topeka Capital-Journal*. But she still couldn't stop drinking.

She died eight months later, much too young at seventy-one, of acute renal failure brought on by alcohol abuse. The pugnacious woman who insisted atop the Albanian Alps that the group dispatch a messenger to British intelligence is buried where she belongs: in a military cemetery at Fort Scott, Kansas. Nolan, who used to steal kisses from her in the "re-creation" room at Camp McCoy, Wisconsin, is still going strong, a grandfather eight times over. The McKenzies' first great-grandchild arrived in October 2012.

The rescue of the 807th MAES from Albania embodied the Allied war effort, good and bad. It was contested, as Lawrence Orville Abbott described the frenzied events near Gjirokastër, with "a savage will." But too much of it was slapdash, plagued by puerile sniping between the Brits and the Americans. Most SOE operatives, Jon Naar asserts, viewed the enterprise as an unwelcome diversion from their mission to help the resistance expel the Germans. The operation, not unlike the land in which it was conducted, was byzantine and balkanized. Naar and his compadres were especially roiled by what they perceived as the gratuitous interference of FDR and OSS.

Yet like the outcome of the war itself, it's hard to argue with the results. Despite its aggravations, the rescue of the 807th MAES should be seen as a triumph. There were a lot of stirring escapes from the Third Reich. But none demanded more of its protagonists or of the Anglo–American–resistance partnership. Against all odds, everyone made it, a testament to the tenacity of the escapees, especially thirteen young women.

It was *Argo* three and a half decades before *Argo*. The 807th's *furtuna* became the Allies' *fortuna*.

The past is like a fog, Herman Wouk has written. "Clutch at it and it wisps through your fingers."

All these years later, the plight of the passengers on Army Aircraft 42-68809 remains mired in intrigue. They took off in fog, flew through a squall, crash-landed in rain, tramped around mountains in sleet and snow, and after it all ended, watched their superiors foist a cloud of silence over their heroics.

That same cloud obscures the preternatural courage of the people who helped them escape, whether they were Albanian resistance leaders, ordinary villagers, or no-holds-barred special ops saboteurs.

It's never too late to salute heroes—or in this case, especially, heroines. The U.S. government should figure out ways to extol the nurses, medics, and airmen, as well as those people who put their lives on the line to save thirty young Americans from a Hitler stalag or firing squad. Thanks to gutsy members of the Albanian *Popullit*, *Fashizmit* was vanquished. It took too long, but the Albanian people are now free.

The American medical team got lost while braving a storm to patch up wounded Tommies in the British Eighth Army. A host of British soldiers then risked everything to rescue the Yanks. In recognition of this mutual valor, perhaps the U.S. and British governments should establish a Gavan B. Duffy Medal, to acknowledge individuals from both countries who have gone to extraordinary lengths to strengthen the "special relationship." It is, after all, despite its warts, among the most important bonds in history.

Only one of the marooned Americans whom Duffy helped rescue is still with us: ninety-one-year-old medic Harold Hayes, who now resides in an assisted-living home in Medford, Oregon. The sergeant who glimpsed the Nazi barrage in Berat at dawn on November 15, 1943, and pronounced it "the Fourth of July in Technicolor" remains sharp as a firecracker.

As Hayes and his friends pounded up and down Balkan mountains, they vowed that if the Lord got them out of their mess, they weren't gonna grieve Him no more. Somewhere in southern Albania, the spiritual's sad and sweet refrain might still be echoing through a valley.

TIME LINE

November 8, 1943   The C-53 crash lands in Albania near Elbasan; Partisan leader Hasan Jina comes to the rescue.

November 12   The Americans arrive in Berat after a three-day march and meet Kostig Steffa, their new Partisan leader.

November 15   The Germans attack Berat. As they flee, the Americans scatter in two groups; three nurses get separated and are left behind.

November 18   The two groups reunite in the hills, but the three nurses remain in a Berat farmhouse.

November 19   The Americans send a message alerting British forces in Albania to their predicament.

November 22	The Americans survive a blizzard climbing the 8,500-foot-high Mount Tomorrit.
November 23	British SOE captain Victor Smith's message reaches the Americans.
November 27	The Americans meet Victor Smith in Lovdar.
December 1	Escorted by Victor Smith, the Americans arrive at British SOE mission headquarters at Krushove.
December 2	The Americans meet SOE's Major Palmer, Lieutenant Duffy, and Sergeant Bell.
December 3	OSS Captain Lloyd Smith's first attempt to reach Albania.
December 5	OSS Captain Smith's second attempt to reach Albania.
December 7	OSS Captain Lloyd Smith finally arrives in Albania at SOE's coastal base, Seaview.
December 8	Duffy and the Americans leave Krushove; Lieutenant John Hamilton and the *Yankee* are ordered not to leave Bari so they can retrieve the party at any moment.
December 12	President Roosevelt telephones SOE Captain Jon Naar in Cairo from U.S.S. *Iowa* in mid-Atlantic.
December 14	Duffy and the Americans climb Mount Nermerska and arrive in Shepr, where Major Tilman and Corporal Williamson are waiting.

December 18	OSS Captain Lloyd Smith and his guides leave for Kuc.
December 20	Thrasher and Baggs ask Duffy to request an air rescue; Duffy declines.
December 21	Duffy relents, allowing the pilots to send a radio message requesting an air rescue.
December 24	Duffy and the group arrive in Doksat near Gjirokastër and the abandoned Italian airstrip.
December 25	The party spends Christmas Day in Doksat.
December 26	The Germans move heavy armor into Gjirokastër, jeopardizing the air rescue attempt.
December 29	The attempted air rescue goes awry.
December 31	Duffy and the group flee Doksat; the group spends New Year's Eve at Saraghinishte.
January 2, 1944	Captain Lloyd Smith, at Dhermi, sends three sets of guides inland to search for the Americans; Duffy sends Steffa, Thrasher, and Albanian guides ahead to survey the trail.
January 4	Duffy and the group cross the Devoll River and arrive in Midhar.
January 5	Duffy and the group arrive in Golem; Captain Lloyd Smith arrives in Vuno.
January 6	Duffy and the group hike through a blizzard and rendezvous with Captain Lloyd Smith outside of Kuç. They continue to Kalarat.

January 7	Steffa leaves the group. Duffy and Smith lead the group on the final push toward Seaview.
January 8	The group climbs the summit of Dukati Mountain and arrives at Seaview. Hamilton's *Yankee* arrives after midnight; Duffy and the group climb aboard.
January 9	The *Yankee* arrives in Bari Harbor about 1:30 p.m.; the group is greeted by 807th colleagues and a bevy of photographers. The members are immediately interrogated by intelligence officers.
February 3	Lloyd Smith, now a major, arrives at Sea Elephant and begins working on Operation Underdone—the rescue of the three nurses in Berat. Tare Shyti is commissioned to wire fake credentials.
February 16–19	Associated Press correspondent Hal Boyle's version of the escape of the original twenty-seven appears in American newspapers, along with photographs of the nurses showing off their beat-up boots.
February 26	German patrols are spotted; Seaview and Sea Elephant are evacuated; Smith makes his way to Dukat with Cooky.
March 14	Smith receives a radio message instructing him that if he cannot get the nurses out of Albania in the next thirty days he is to return to Bari.
March 15	Two Albanians come to the nurses' farmhouse with material and instruct the nurses to begin making peasant dresses.

March 18	The disguised nurses leave Berat in a car with Shyti; they're followed by a truck of Albanian soldiers; the caravan takes them within a day's hike of Dukati Mountain.
March 19	The group rendezvous with Smith and Cooky near Dukat. That night, Smith takes the nurses down the Valona-Dukat road.
March 20	The group rests in a house near Dukati Mountain. Just before midnight they start climbing the mountain.
March 21	The group reaches the summit about noon and arrives at Seaview that evening. At midnight an Italian motorboat, helmed by an OSS pilot, picks up Smith and the nurses.
March 22	Thirteen hours after boarding the boat, the nurses and Smith arrive in Otranto, Italy.
March 23	The nurses are taken to the hospital in Bari.

—COMPILED BY CAMERON SMITH HOWARD

ACKNOWLEDGMENTS

I first learned about the spectacular escape of American nurses and medics trapped in Nazi-occupied Albania while researching *Assignment to Hell,* my 2012 book about World War II correspondents. Hal Boyle of the Associated Press, one of the five journalists whose work I celebrated, had a near-exclusive in early 1944 about the medical team's crash-landing and miraculous escape. Boyle's story floored me; when I first saw the clip in 2009 I scribbled in the margin: "Whoa. This is a book!"

Getting the Americans out of those mountains took ingenuity and grit: from the castaways themselves, from Allied intelligence operatives, and from the Partisan guerrillas and impoverished peasants, most Muslim, but Roman Catholic and Orthodox families, too, who risked everything to feed and hide sworn enemies of the Reich.

Like Boyle, I found the entire episode irresistible. So, fortunately, did a lot of other people who proved invaluable on this project.

At the top of the list is Cameron Smith Howard, who tracked down information about the saga's principals, spotlighted key milestones (a movie buff, she called them "juicy bits"), critiqued various drafts of the manuscript, and compiled a time line. Her parents, both die-hard Dookies, as is Cameron, claim that she was not named after Duke University's notorious basketball arena, but I'm skeptical. Remember the way Grant Hill attacked the rim? That's the way Cameron does research.

The wondrous Jon Naar, ninety-three and still going strong, who seven decades ago got yelled at by President Roosevelt (and how many people still alive can say that?), provided invaluable insights into the history of SOE and OSS and was kind enough to incorporate those thoughts into the manuscript. He writes as nimbly as he once skulked behind Rommel's lines in Egypt. You can admire Jon's brilliant photography at www.jonnaar.com.

The folks at the Library of Congress, as always, came through in the clutch. Old pal David Kelly, now retired from the library, shoved me in the right direction for the fourth time. His colleague Gary Johnson, a World War II buff who works in the library's newspapers and periodicals room, did yeoman work on my behalf. It took Gary only minutes to locate the 1947 *True Comics* issue with the "Balkan Escape" strip. Impressive.

Their counterparts at the National Archives and National Archives II in College Park, Maryland, were invaluable, too. Amy Schmidt and her colleagues patiently guided me through II's voluminous files on the OSS.

The people at the British National Archives at Kew Gardens were also great. Hugh Alexander helped me pick out photographs from SOE's remarkable collection and went to great lengths to dig out the shot from Garry Duffy's personnel files. Just seeing the visage of the young Duffy made my trip to London worthwhile. So did running into SOE scholar Steve Kippax, who generously shared his files and insights. Samuel Shearin at the Air Force Historical Research Agency also did yeoman work in digging up photos.

Britta Granrud, the curator of the Women in Memorial Service to America Foundation, kindly put together a disk of WIMSA's various interviews with and materials from 807th principals.

The children and grandchildren of the nurses, medics, and airmen should also be singled out for special thanks. Clint Abbott and Phyllis McKenzie both spent hours digging into family archives and unearthed incredible stuff, and were also kind enough to fact-check the manuscript. Phyllis's father, Nolan McKenzie, and son, Eric McKenzie, were also invaluable. Agnes Jensen's daughter, Karen, spent time with me on the phone early in my research. Dick Lebo's daughter, Gayle Yost, became an e-mail pal, as did Jean Rutkowski's daughter, Lee Whitson. Both provided wonderful letters from their respective parents' papers.

Leka Bezhani, the grandson of the great Tare Shyti, the rescuer of the final three nurses trapped in Berat, provided terrific insights into his family's heritage and Albania's troubled past. So did Peter Lucas, the Boston journalistic institution who's written two books on Albania's past, including a history of the OSS in Albania, and accompanied Agnes Jensen Mangerich to Albania in 1995.

Colleague and nautical buff Brian Sailer furnished a description Sterling Hayden's getaway boat, the *Yankee*. Colleague and wrestling buff Neal Urwitz furnished the term "grappler" to describe Lloyd Smith. Old pal Steve Harper, also a proud alum of Warren (Pennsylvania) Area High School, Class of 1972, provided Italian translations.

Brent Howard, my editor at New American Library Penguin, loves World War II history as much as I do. No writer of popular history could ever find a better friend or a more conscientious editor.

But as always, the ultimate thanks go to Elizabeth, Allyson, Andrew, and Abigail, who were amazingly helpful and patient on number four and let Dad go to Europe solo this time.

BIBLIOGRAPHY

UNPUBLISHED SOURCES

Abbott, Clint W., son of Sgt. Lawrence O. Abbott. Telephone and e-mail interviews, April–August 2012.

Abbott, Sgt. Lawrence O. Mementos and materials from personal archives provided by his son, Clint.

Bell, Herbert John, Sgt., personnel file, SOE archives, British National Archives, Kew Gardens, London.

Bezhani, Leka, grandson of Albanian patriot hero Tare Shyti. E-mail interviews, November 2012–January 2013. Mementos and materials from family archives.

Boyle, Hal, World War II scrapbook compiled by his sister-in-law, Monica Murphy Boyle, and generously lent by her son Ed, Hal's nephew.

Curtis, Karen Mangerich, daugter of Lt. Agnes Jensen Mangerich. Interviewed by telephone, August 2012.

Duffy, Capt. (formerly Lt.) Gavan B. Various after-action reports submitted December 1943 and January 1944 describing efforts to escape

Albania with American party, SOE papers, British National Archives, Kew Gardens, London.

———. Personnel and medal commendation files, SOE papers, British National Archives, Kew Gardens, London.

Foster, Terry, researcher, U.S. Army Military Research Center, Carlisle Barracks, Pennsylvania. Interviewed by telephone and e-mail, April–June 2012.

Hayes, Sgt. Harold, Medford, Oregon, the 807th MAES's sole survivor. Telephone interviews, August–September 2012.

Hayes, Harold, letter to Larry O. Abbott, January 17, 1961, courtesy of Clint Abbott.

———, interview in Women in Memorial Service to America (WIMSA) archives, Arlington, Virginia.

Kelly, David, former researcher, Library of Congress. Interviewed by phone and e-mail, May–June 2012.

Kippax, Steve, British SOE expert. Interviewed in London, November–December 2012 and via e-mail December 2012–January 2013. Provided voluminous SOE documents.

Komor, Valerie, archivist, Associated Press. Interviewed in New York, April 2010, and by phone and e-mail, 2010–2011.

Kuhn, Betsy, interview with Agnes Jensen Mangerich, conducted October 31, 1995, in WIMSA archives, Arlington, Virginia.

Layzell, Alastair, British television documentary producer. Interviewed in London, November–December 2012, and via e-mail, August 2012–January 2013.

Mangerich, Agnes Jensen, March 24, 1992 interview, in WIMSA archives, Arlington, Virginia.

———. Memorial materials from 2010 service, WIMSA files, Arlington, Virginia.

McKenzie, Eric, grandson of Lt. Lois Watson McKenzie. Interviewed via mail and e-mail, March 2012–June 2012.

McKenzie, Lt. Lois. Biographical memoir prepared for February 1991 forum at Washburn University on wartime nursing. In WIMSA files, Arlington, Virginia, and provided by her daughter Phyllis.

———. Shorter biographic memoir written in 1983. In WIMSA files, Arlington, Virginia, and provided by her daughter Phyllis.

McKenzie, Nolan, widower of Lt. Lois Watson McKenzie. Interviewed by phone and via mail and e-mail through his grandson Eric McKenzie, March–June 2012. Provided mementos and materials from personal archives.

McKenzie, Phyllis, daughter of Lt. Lois Watson McKenzie. Interviewed by telephone June–August 2012, and via e-mail, June 2012–January 2013. Provided mementos and materials from her parents' personal archives.

McManus, John C., World War II historian and professor at the Missouri University of Science and Technology, Rolla, Missouri. Interviewed via e-mail, March–June 2012.

Naar, Jon, former SOE major and head of Albanian B8 section, Special Operations Mediterranean in Cairo and Bari, 1943–1944. Interviewed in person and by telephone and e-mail, September 2012–March 2013.

———. Unpublished memoir, *Time to Tell*, and other mementos and photographs from personal archives.

Office of Strategic Services (OSS), various memoranda and histories of Albanian and Balkan resistance movement, monthly reports from Mediterranean desk, and various after-action reports, National Archives II, College Park, Maryland.

Rutkowski, Lt. Jean. Undated letter to daughter, Lee Whitson, about her experiences in the 807th MAES, Lee Whitson's personal files.

Smith, Lt. Col. (formerly Capt. and Maj.) Lloyd. Various after-action reports submitted December 1943–April 1944 describing efforts to rescue American party from Albania, OSS files, National Archives II, College Park, Maryland.

———. Handwritten "Report of Mission of Evacuation, American Rescue Party, Period Nov. 30, 1943, to January 9, 1944." WIMSA files, Arlington, Virginia.

———. Personnel and medal commendation files, OSS papers, National Archives II, College Park, Maryland.

Special Operations Executive (SOE), various Albanian and Balkan resistance reports and analyses, various monthly updates from British liaison officers and others, British National Archives, Kew Gardens, London.

Whitson, Lee, daughter of Lt. Jean Rutkowski. Interviewed by phone and e-mail, December 2012–January 2013. Provided materials from her late mother's personal files.

Yost, Gayle Lebo, daughter of Sgt. Dick Lebo. Interviewed via e-mail, December 2012–January 2013. Provided letter about her father's World War II record she sent to the *Harrisburg Patriot-News*.

PUBLISHED SOURCES

Books

Abbott, Lawrence O., and Abbott, Clinton W. *Out of Albania—From the Memoirs of Lawrence O. Abbott, A True Account of a WW II Underground Rescue Mission.* USA: Lulu Press, 2010.

Ambrose, Stephen E. *The Victors: Eisenhower and His Boys: The Men of World War II.* New York: Simon & Schuster, 1998.

———. *The Wild Blue: The Men and Boys Who Flew the B-24s Over Germany.* New York: Simon & Schuster, 2001.

Amery, Julian. *Sons of the Eagle: A Study in Guerrilla War.* London: Macmillan & Co. Ltd., 1948.

Associated Press. *Breaking News: How the Associated Press Has Covered War, Peace, and Everything Else,* with a foreword by David Halberstam. New York: Princeton Architectural Press, 2007.

Atkinson, Rick. *An Army at Dawn: The War in North Africa, 1942–1943.* New York: Henry Holt and Company, 2002.

———. *The Day of Battle: The War in Sicily and Italy, 1943–1944.* New York: Henry Holt and Company, 2007.

Bailey, Roderick. *The Wildest Province: SOE in the Land of the Eagle.* London: Jonathan Cape, 2009.

Bailey, Ronald H., and the editors of Time-Life Books. *Partisans and Guerrillas.* Alexandria, VA: Time-Life Books, 1979.

Boyle, Hal, comp. *Help, Help! Another Day!* New York: Associated Press, 1969.

Breur, William B. *Unexplained Mysteries of World War II.* New York: John Wiley & Sons, 1997.

Brokaw, Tom. *The Greatest Generation Speaks: Letters and Reflections.* Toronto and New York: Random House, 1999.

Conn, Stetson, general ed. *United States Army in World War II.* Washington, D.C.: Center of Military History, 1961.

Cowley, Robert, ed. *No End Save Victory: Perspectives on World War II.* New York: G. P. Putnam, 2001.

Dunnigan, James F., and Albert A. Nofi. *Dirty Little Secrets of World War II.* New York: William Morrow and Company, 1994.

Ellis, John. *Brute Force: Allied Strategy and Tactics in the Second World War.* New York: Viking, 1990.

Fessler, Diane Burke. *No Time for Fear: Voices of American Nurses in World War II.* East Lansing, MI: Michigan State University Press, 1996.

Flight Nurses Association, Inc. *Legends of the Flight Nurses.* Series of biographical sketches maintained online by legendsofflightnurses.org.

Ford, Kirk, Jr. *OSS and the Yugoslav Resistance, 1943–1945.* College Station: Texas A&M University Press, 2000.

Freeman, Gregory A. *The Forgotten 500: The Untold Story of the Men Who Risked All for the Greatest Rescue Mission of World War II.* New York: NAL Caliber, 2007.

Groom, Winston. *1942: The Year That Tried Men's Souls.* New York: Atlantic Monthly Press, 2005.

Hart, B. H. Liddel. *History of the Second World War.* New York: DaCapo Press, 1970.

Keegan, John. *The Battle for History: Re-fighting World War II.* New York, Vintage Books, 1996.

———. *The Second World War.* New York: Viking Penguin, 1990.

Kemp, Peter. *No Colours or Crest.* London: Cassell, 1958.

Infield, Glenn B. *Disaster at Bari.* New York: Bantam Books, 1988.

Leary, William M. *Fueling the Fires of Resistance: Army Air Forces Special Operations in the Balkans During World War II.* Washington, D.C.: Air Force History and Museums Program, 1995.

Lindsay, Franklin. *Beacons in the Night: With the OSS and Tito's Partisans in Wartime Yugoslavia.* Palo Alto: Stanford University Press, 1996.

Lineberry, Cate. *The Secret Rescue: An Untold Story of American Nurses and Medics Behind Enemy Lines.* New York: Little Brown and Company, 2013.

Lucas, Peter. *The O.S.S. in World War II Albania: Covert Operations and Collaborations with Communist Partisans.* Jefferson, N.C.: McFarland & Company, Inc., 2007.

———. *Rumpalla: Rummaging Through Albania.* Boston: Xlibris, 2002.

MacCloskey, Brig. Gen. Monro, USAF (ret.). *Secret Air Missions.* New York: Richards Rosen Press, Inc., 1966.

Mangerich, Agnes Jensen, as told to Evelyn M. Monahan and Rosemary L. Neidel. *Albanian Escape: The True Story of U.S. Army Nurses Behind Enemy Lines.* Lexington: University Press of Kentucky, 1999.

Marmullaku, Ramadan. *Albania and the Albanians.* London: Archon Books, 1975.

Miller, Donald L. *Masters of the Air: America's Bomber Boys Who Fought the Air War Against Nazi Germany.* New York: Simon & Schuster, 2006.

————. (original text by Henry Steele Commager). *The Story of World War II*. New York: Touchstone, 2011.

Monahan, Evelyn M., and Neidel-Greenlee, Rosemary. *And if I Perish: Frontline U.S. Army Nurses in World War II*. New York: Knopf Doubleday Publishing Group, 2003.

Nichols, David, ed. *Ernie's War: The Best of Ernie Pyle's War Dispatches*. New York: Random House, 1986.

Persico, Joseph E. *Roosevelt's Secret War: FDR and World War II Espionage*. New York: Random House, 2002.

Quayle, Sir Anthony. *A Time to Speak*. London: Barrie & Jenkins, 1992.

Ruches, Pyrrhus. *Albania's Captives*. Chicago: Argonaut, 1965.

Šelhaus, Edi. *Evasion and Repatriation: Slovene Partisans and Rescued American Airmen in World War II*. Manhattan, KS: Sunflower University Press, 1995.

Skendk, Stavro, ed. *Albania*. New York: Praeger, 1956.

Smiley, David. *Albanian Assignment*. London: Chatto & Windus, The Hogarth Press, 1985.

Thruelsen, Richard, and Elliott Arnold. *Mediterranean Sweep: Air Stories from El Alamein to Rome*. New York: Duell, Sloan and Pearce, 1945.

Tobin, James. *Ernie Pyle's War: America's Eyewitness to World War II*. New York: The Free Press (a division of Simon & Schuster), 1997.

Vickers, Miranda. *The Albanians: Modern History*. London/New York: I. B. Taurus & Co. Ltd, 1999.

Vickers, Miranda, and James Pettifer. *Albania from Anarchy to a Balkan Identity*. New York: New York University Press, 1997.

Ward, Geoffrey C., and Ken Burns. *The War: An Intimate History*. New York: Alfred A. Knopf, 2007.

Weatherford, Doris. *American Women During World War II: An Encyclopedia*. New York: Castle Books, 2009.

Wilmot, Chester. *The Struggle for Europe*. London: The Reprint Society, 1952.

Winnifrith, Tom, ed. *Perspectives on Albania*. London: Macmillan, 1992.

Wright, Mike. *What They Didn't Teach You About World War II*. Novato, CA: Presidio Press, 1998.

Magazines, Journals, and Specialty Publications

Air Force: The Official Service Journal of the U.S. Army Air Forces
Collier's

DDA Magazine (Dutch)
German Anti-Guerrilla Operations in the Balkans (1941–1944—CMH Publication)
Illinois Central Magazine
Lake County's (Florida) *Golden Lifestyles*
Providence (Hospital) *News*
True Comics
Women's Quarterly, A Supplement to The Daily Commercial (Leesburg, Florida)
Yank: The Army Weekly

Newspapers

Atlanta Constitution
Baltimore Sun
Bethesda (Maryland) *Almanac*
Big Rapids (Michigan) *Pioneer*
Boston Globe
Brockton (Massachusetts) *Enterprise*
Chicago Daily Tribune
Chicago Sun
Chicago Times
Dayton Daily News
Detroit Free Press
Detroit News
Grand Rapids Press
Hartford Courant
Kalamazoo (Michigan) *Gazette*
Leesburg (Florida) *Daily Commercial*
Liverpool (UK) *Daily Post*
London Daily Mail
Newago County (Michigan) *Times-Indicator*
New York Sun
New York Times
Orlando Sentinel
Providence Journal
San Antonio Express-News
The Stars and Stripes
Times of London

Topeka Capital-Journal
Washington Post
Washington Times

Broadcast

Brief film of American party arriving in Bari, Italy, January 9, 1944, in files of National Archives II, College Park, Maryland.

Web sites

www.afhra.af.mil
www.archives.gov/
www.loc.gov/
www.nationalarchives.gov.uk/
www.warwingsart.com/12thAirForce
www.rtbot.net/Albanian_Resistance-Of_World_War_II
www.pacificbattleship.com/page/battleship_of_presidents
www.warlinks.com
www.fdrlibrary.marist.edu
www.legendsofflightnurses.org
www.nationalmuseum.af.mil
www.ibiblio.org/hyperwar/ETO/East/Balkans
www.huntleyandpalmers.com
www.mountaineersbooks.org
www.imdb.com/name/nm0001330/bio
www.academia.edu/2330113/THE_MOST_SECRET_LIST_OF_SOE_
AGENTS
www.archives.gov/research/arc/ww2/navy-casualties/south-dakota.html
www.globalsecurity.org/intell/ops/albania.htm

NOTES

PROLOGUE:
SAVING THE "FLOWER OF AMERICAN WOMANHOOD"

The information about FDR's November–December 1943 itinerary comes from the day-to-day chronology available through the Franklin D. Roosevelt Presidential Library, at www.fdrlibrary.marist.edu. The *Iowa* bathtub story comes from www.pacificbattleship.com/page/battleship_ of_presidents.

FDR's patrician fascination with espionage was documented in Joseph Persico's *Roosevelt's Secret War: FDR and World War II Espionage*, pp. 4–5. The information on FDR's Cairo "mole," OSS major Harry T. Fultz, comes from interviews with Jon Naar.

The *Iowa*'s ship's position information was provided by the FDR library, via a December 2012 e-mail.

Jon Naar's recollections of his conversations with FDR and Major Philip Leake were recounted in various telephone interviews in the fall of 2012, over lunch at Union Station in Washington, D.C., on November 23, 2012, and through a series of e-mail exchanges in late 2012 and early 2013. The long quote from Naar describing the FDR call, as well as his recollection of Leake's reaction, comes from his as-yet-unpublished memoir, tentatively titled *Time to Tell*.

The great British satirist P. G. Wodehouse was a proud alumnus of Leake's South London public school, Dulwich.

CHAPTER 1:
LOST IN THE FOG OF WAR

Lois Watson McKenzie's recollections of the fateful flight were recorded in two self-penned documents that were provided by her daughter Phyllis McKenzie; they're also available in the archives of the Women in Military Service for America Memorial Foundation archives (WIMSA). Agnes Jensen Mangerich's recollections of the flight come from her *Albanian Escape*, pp. 9–19, and through two lengthy interviews, one conducted in 1991 and the other in 1995, by interviewer Betsy Kuhn, both available in the WIMSA archives. The "sparks" metaphor comes from Lawrence Orville Abbott's *Out of Albania*, p. 13.

The story of the medic "shaking like a leaf" comes from an interview Jens gave to the *Bethesda Almanac*, published on July 4, 1990, p. 1; the article is also available in the WIMSA archives.

The information about all the remarkable subterfuge involved in the episode comes from Jon Naar and various SOE and OSS documents, available, respectively, from the British National Archives in Kew, London, and the U.S. National Archives II, College Park, Maryland. The information on the *Argo*-like quality of the rescue comes from Major Lloyd Smith's after-action analyses in the OSS files at National Archives II (some of which were also highlighted in Jens's *Albanian Escape*), from interviews with Leka Bezhani, the grandson of Albanian hero Tare Shyti, and from Peter Lucas's book on the OSS in Albania.

Tare Shyti was clearly an Albanian "patriot" who aligned himself with the Allied cause. He was not, however, a "Partisan," which has come to be synonymous with "Communist guerrilla fighter." For purposes of this book, all Partisans were patriots but not all patriots were Partisans.

The *Casablanca* "stretcher bearer" story and much of the information on the Allies' Italian campaign comes from the great Rick Atkinson's *Day of Battle*, p. 262. The Ernie Pyle "tough old gut" line comes from a column Pyle wrote in November 1943 from the Italian front, which I also used in my *Assignment to Hell*, p. 217.

The information on the British Eighth's November 1943 Italian offensive comes from the British Fourth Armoured's battle history at www.war links.com.

The Garry Duffy biographical information comes from his SOE personnel files at the British National Archives, from Roderick Bailey's *The Wildest Province*, pp. 58–60, and from Jon Naar's recollections. The story about Duffy's determination to "win" the race to rescue the nurses comes from David Smiley's *Albanian Assignment*, p. 104.

The background information on Naar comes from Naar himself, particularly our conversation over lunch on November 23, 2012, and his critique of the manuscript. The information on the Albanian patriots comes from Mangerich and Abbott and from a series of e-mails from Leka Bezhani sent in November and December of 2012.

The information on Lloyd Smith comes from OSS files, including his personnel file and medal commendation file, his after-action report for OSS, and from Mangerich's *Albanian Escape*, which highlighted a number of his after-action reports. The wrestling insight comes from friend and colleague Neal Urwitz.

CHAPTER 2:
FURTUNA OVER THE IONIAN

The Italian translations in the book come courtesy of old friend Stephen Knox Harper, Esq., who knows two more languages than I do. Mangerich and Abbott both have detailed accounts of the 807th's preflight activities in their respective books, pp. 9–10 for Mangerich, pp. 9–11 for Abbott. Lois Watson McKenzie also has a detailed account in her 1991 recollection, including a reference to the B-25 crew, which is also available in the WIMSA archives.

The information on the 807th's Bowman Field, North African, and Bari experiences comes from McKenzie's two autobiographical papers, Jean Rutkowski's letter to her daughter, Lee Whitson, which Lee generously provided, and *The History of the 807th MAES* by Dorothy White Errair, highlighted in Errair's material in the Legends of the Flight Nurses of World War II Web site, www.legendsofflightnurses.org. The 21 and New York City leave stories come from Jean Rutkowski's letter. Information on the 807th's Catania experience comes from Lois McKenzie's papers and personal photographs, generously provided by her daughter Phyllis, and from Rutkowski's letter.

The Sicilian campaign background on Catania and Montgomery comes from Atkinson's *Day of Battle*, pp. 127–30.

The Grottaglie reference comes from Abbott, p. 9; descriptions of the attire of 807th members that fateful morning comes from Lois McKenzie's papers, Mangerich pp. 9–11, and Abbott pp. 9–11.

The information on the history of medical flight evacuation comes from the article "Wings for the Wounded," by Lieutenant Colonel Richard L. Meiling, which appeared in the December 1943 issue of *Air Force: The Official Service Journal of the U.S. Army Air Forces*, p. 53. The statistics on medical flight evacuation training and the casualty rate come from an October 6, 2001, article in the *Dayton* (Ohio) *Daily News*, entitled "WWII Flight Nurses Gather, Reminisce," p. 1-B; the article is part of the Errair materials in the Legends of the Flight Nurses site. The squadron breakdown figures comes from an article entitled "Angels on Board" that appeared in the January 21, 2002, edition of *DDA Magazine* (a Dutch periodical), pp. 11–12, which is also included in the Legends of the Flight Nurses site.

McKenzie's Bowman Field quote and other training memories come from her 1991 Washburn University nurses' forum paper, p. 4.

The *Santa Elena* recollections come from a telephone interview with Harold Hayes, conducted August 12, 2012, and from Rutkowski's letter. Information on the 807th's experiences in North Africa comes from McKenzie's Washburn paper, p. 5, and Rutkowski's letter. The success of medical flight evacuation statistics comes from the Meiling *Air Force* article, p. 22.

The information on Corporal Gilbert Hornsby comes from Abbott, p. 9, as does the quote about the efficacy of C-47 transports. The C-47/C-53 data comes from the U.S. Air Force museum's online history, www.nationalmuseum.af.mil.

The Thompson machine gun and gin rummy recollections appear in Abbott, pp. 10–11. Jens's memories of sitting next to the radio set and Elna Schwant appear in *Albanian Escape*, pp. 11–19. The Simpson reference appears in Jens's book, p. 10.

The aircraft serial number appears in the official USAAF document highlighted on p. 51 of Jens's book. The "fear and panic" line appears in Jens's book, p. 12.

The Yarbrough instructions appear in Jens's book, p. 13. The "translucent" description of Jens's eyes appears in the 1990 *Bethesda Almanac* article. Jens's recollections of her Michigan childhood and nurse's training appear in the interviews conducted in 1991 and 1995, WIMSA archives. The reference to Jens's parents fretting over her dangerous duties appears in *Albanian Escape*, p. 211.

The "nothing, nothing, nothing" quote is from Jens's 1995 Kuhn interview, p. 3. The official flight log information appears in Jens's book, pp. 14–15.

McKenzie's waterspout recollection appears in her 1991 Washburn paper, p. 8. Much of the information on Lois's childhood, including the various boyfriend stories and the wonderful "hellhole" exchange, comes from a series of e-mails sent by her daughter Phyllis in the summer and fall of 2012, as well as Lois's own papers.

The information about Harry Dee Watson's job came from the *Illinois Central Magazine*, March 1944, p. 23, in the WISMA archives. The banana peel quote comes from Lois McKenzie's Washburn paper, p. 2, as does the "re-creation" quote, p. 3.

Schwant's "Mountains?" query appears in Jens's book, p. 15. Abbott's waterspout story appears in his book, p. 11. As mentioned in Cate Lineberry's *The Secret Rescue*, p. 49, medic Harold Hayes recalled that it was Focke-Wulf Fw190s chasing them, not Messerschmitts. McKenzie's observation about no panicky chatter appears in her Washburn paper, p. 8.

Abbott's recollections of the "real airfield" exchange appear in his book, p. 13. The Bowman Field missing parachutes story appears in McKenzie's Washburn paper, p. 8.

The Bob Owen–German pistol story appears in Abbott, p. 15.

CHAPTER 3:
THE CRASH-LANDING—*AMERICANO! AMERICANO!*

The "cough and spit" line comes from Abbott, p. 15. Most of the background on the Abbott family and the history of western Michigan comes from a series of e-mails from and telephone conversations with Clint Abbott, Orville's son, in the summer and fall of 2012.

Jens's "never get out" quote is from the 1990 *Bethesda Almanac* piece. Thrasher's buckle-up quote comes from Jens's 1995 Kuhn interview, p. 4.

Abbott's facial muscles reference appears in his book, p. 16, as does his recollection of Shumway the broad jumper and the "pretty" three-point landing.

The "mire" comment and the "any good landing" comment comes from Jens's 1995 interview with Kuhn, pp. 3–4. Abbott's "silent and brooding" observation comes from his book, p. 17.

The descriptions of the native Albanians and their reaction to the Americans' surprise arrival comes from a combination of Abbott (pp. 15–23), McKenzie (both papers), and Mangerich (pp. 21–28).

The "Roosh-a" comment comes from the McKenzie Washburn paper, p. 11. Thrasher's epithet comes from Jon Naar's unpublished memoir, chapter 2.

The spelling of Albanian names and words in English is an inexact science. Writer Peter Lucas, who is of Albanian descent, spelled the name of the Albanian Partisan leader "Hasan" (with one "s") "Jina" (with a "J"). Jens and Abbott spelled his first name with two "s's" and his last name with a "G." Since Peter is more familiar with the culture, I went with his version.

Hasan's "never mind" tic first appears in Abbott's book, p. 20; the "Germans do not take you" on p. 21.

The "oldest still-spoken language" references come from Peter Lucas's *The OSS in World War II Albania*, p. 15. The various Albanian terms come from Miranda Vickers's *Modern History of Albania*, p. ix, and from Lucas's *Rumpalla*, pp. 21–22. The Caesar reference comes from Lucas's *OSS*, pp. 15–16. The other Roman historical references come from Lucas's *Rumpalla*, p. 126.

The George Kastrioti information comes from Appendix A in Vickers's *Modern History*, p. 581. The "Sons of the Eagle" reference comes from Lucas's *Rumpalla*, p. 21. The Gibbon references come from Miranda Vickers and James Pettifer's *Albania: From Anarchy to a Balkan Identity*, p. 1. The information on Albania's break with the Ottoman Empire in 1912 comes from Lucas's *OSS*, p. 17.

The Gheg-Tosk description comes from Julian Amery's *Sons of the Eagle*, p. 13. The Noli information comes from Lucas's *OSS*, p. 17, as well as Vickers's *Modern History* Appendix A, p. 581. The Soviet Union's lack of interest in Albania comes from Vickers's *Modern History*, p. 145; the King Zog uniform story from the same book, p. 124.

The Mussolini-Zog information comes from Vickers's *Modern History* Appendix A, p. 582. The Good Friday invasion story comes from Lucas's *Rumpalla,* p. 126. The "foreclose the mortgage quote" comes from "History," an official SOE history of wartime Albania located in the British National Archives, Kew Gardens, London.

The Mussolini newspaper reference comes from p. 616 of Vickers's *Modern History* Appendix A; the Tomori legend from p. 618.

Lucas's description of Hoxha as a "pocket-sized Stalin" appears on p. 128 of *Rumpalla*. The "professor" reference to Hoxha comes from Smiley's book, p. 56. Jon Naar shared SOE's assessment of Hoxha via interviews and his critique of the original manuscript.

The Bajraktari and Peza references come from Smiley, pp. 145–46.

The Churchill Albanian quote is referenced in Naar's unpublished memoir, chapter 11, p. 1. The size of Albania analogy comes from an article entitled "German Anti-Guerrilla Activities in the Balkans, 1941–1944," p. 6; it's available from www.ibiblio.org/hyperwar/ETO/East/Balkans.

The Hoxha-Runi story comes from Lucas's *Rumpalla*, p. 122, and from two telephone interviews with Lucas in the fall of 2012. The story about corn and tobacco hanging from the rafters comes from McKenzie's Washburn paper, p. 11.

Abbott and Mangerich don't agree on when and how the C-53 was torched. Jens says right away; Orville says it took two days and two attempts before it finally burned. I went with Abbott's account, since he was part of the posse that set fire to the plane and wrote about it less than two years after the incident occurred. There was also disagreement as to exactly when the castaways were told about British officers being stationed on the ground in Albania. McKenzie, Jens, and Abbott all said the Hasan (and later Steffa) informed them fairly early on that there were Brits in Albania, although it's unclear that the Americans understood from the outset that the Brits were intelligence officers dedicated, in part, to helping downed Allied airmen. As referenced in Lineberry's book and in his interview in the WIMSA files. Hayes believes that they weren't told about the presence of British officers until several weeks into their ordeal.

Descriptions of the rest of their first day stranded in Albania come from a compilation of Abbott's book, Jens's book, McKenzie's papers, Rutkowski's letter, and Ann Maness's 1991 interview, also on file at WIMSA. The description of how Albanian corn bread was prepared comes from Rutkowski's letter.

The Çerriku son Faik's story about Shumway and the stretcher comes from Lucas's *Rumpalla*, p. 121. The female guerrillas story comes from Jens's book, pp. 31–32.

The Reich's dependence on Balkan natural resources comes from the "Anti-Guerrilla" article, p. 31.

Much of the information on the Italy-Greek war and its impact on the Reich's war strategy comes from Persico's *Roosevelt's Secret War*, pp. 332–33.

Operation Barbarossa's delay "costing the Germans dearly" comes from Lucas's *Rumpalla*, p. 121. The well-dressed-gentleman story comes from Jens's book, p. 33; his suspected identity and motivation from Lucas's *Rumpalla*, p. 121, and from telephone interviews with Lucas.

The water buffalo dinner story appears in different forms in the recollections of Abbott, Mangerich, McKenzie, and Maness, as well as the book *Mediterranean Sweep*.

CHAPTER 4:
SURREAL HEROES IN BERAT

The face-splashing method of bathing is described on p. 33 of Abbott's book. Jean Rutkowski's peeing-in-the-bushes story comes from a telephone conversation with her daughter, Lee Whitson, on December 27, 2012.

Jens's eavesdropping story with Hasan and Baggs appears in her book, pp. 39–41. The parachute scarves and spirits-improved story comes from Abbott, p. 34.

Jens's recollection of that day's lunch on the trail comes from her book, p. 41.

Much of the Albanian resistance history, including the reference to the forbidden newspaper and the "pronounced difference" quote, comes from Vickers's *Modern History*, pp. 147–48. Abbott and McKenzie both recalled the Americans calling Ballists "Barleys."

The "they were of every age" quote comes from Lucas's *OSS*, pp. 32–33. The Italian casualty figure is referenced in Lucas's *Rumpalla*, p. 120. The Quayle "harnessed together" quote comes from Lucas's *OSS*, p. 34.

The Borova massacre reference comes from an October 4, 2012, telephone conversation with Lucas. The *Ustascha* reference comes from the "Anti-Guerrilla" article, p. 28, and from Jon Naar's manuscript critique.

The missing-galoshes story appears in Jens's book, pp. 41–42. The Tirana banker story comes from the same book, p. 43.

The lovely throat-cutting anecdote comes from onetime Franco defender Peter Kemp's *No Colours or Crest*, p. 104.

The Hasan "not so funny" riff comes from Abbott, p. 38. Jens and Abbott each have a description of how they concealed themselves from the German airfield; Abbott's is on p. 39 of his book; Jens's is on p. 44 of her book.

Abbott's account of the attack on the Berat airfield appears in his book, pp. 41–42. Jens's account appears on pp. 45–46 of her book.

The statistical information on the November 12, 1943, airfield attack comes from a 12th Air Force chronology, available at www.warwingsart.com/12thAirForce.

Their triumphant march into Berat is covered in Jens's book, pp. 47–50, and in Abbott's book, pp. 42–43. The Cruise "pill-roller" line comes from Abbott, p. 43.

Abbott and Jens had different versions of Hasan's departure sequence; again I favored Abbott's, which appears on p. 46 of his book, along with the "pheasants" line. Jens's description of Hasan's departure appears on p. 51 of her book.

Jens's description of their first night in Berat appears in her book, pp. 48–51. Abbott's description of the boys' night out on the town with Chris appears on pp. 46–47. The story of Gino's long-winded speech appears in Abbott, p. 49.

Much of the early SOE history comes from Monroe MacCloskey's *Secret Air Missions*, pp. 16–21, and from a memorandum to me written in January 2013 by Jon Naar.

Descriptions of the castaways' last two days in Berat appears in Jens's book, pp. 53–55, and in Abbott's, pp. 48–49.

CHAPTER 5:
SEPARATION—THE GERMANS ATTACK

Descriptions of the German attack on Berat appear in Jens's book, pp. 54–61, and in Abbott's book, pp. 50–57.

The castaways' escape from Berat via the mountains is covered in Jens's book, pp. 61–66, and in Abbott's, pp. 58–64. "Johnny's" identity is finally revealed on p. 213 of Jens's book.

Jens and Abbott both claim that Seargent J. P. Wolf was with their respective group as they got separated fleeing Berat, which isn't possible, since Jens and Abbott were in different groups. Again, since Abbott was writing so much closer to the actual event, my inclination was to go with his account.

Jens's spectacular account of the BK ambush and the nurses being pressed into emergency duty to patch up the Partisan fighters appears on pp. 65–68 of her book.

The John Kenneth Galbraith quote appears on pp. vii–viii of Franklin Lindsay's *Beacons in the Night*. The Albania "first country" quote appears on p. 1 of "History," the SOE's official history of Albanian Resistance in the British National Archives.

The Leninist uprising reference comes Lindsay, p. ix. Much of the Tito background, including the Himmler quote, comes from Ronald H. Bailey's *Partisans and Guerrillas*, p. 142.

The Mihailovic background, including the "beat them to their knees" quote, comes from Ronald Bailey's book, pp. 115–20. The Maclean "same old slogans" quote comes from the same book, p. 122. The same page holds the Maclean-Churchill exchange, which was verified by Jon Naar, who was stationed with SOM in Cairo at the time of the first and second Cairo conferences, fall 1943.

Churchill's rebuff of Donovan appears in Persico's *Roosevelt's Secret War*, pp. 334–35. Lynne Farish's superb description of Yugoslav history is quoted in Persico, p. 335.

The Kemp quote on Smiley appears on p. 99 of Kemp's *No Colours or Crest*. Kemp's description of Duffy's bomb making as "uncanny" appears in the same book, p. 93.

Smiley's "Calais" quote on Duffy appears on p. 14 of *Albanian Assignment*; the food reference is on p. 26. The Duffy French deficiency story appears on p. 54 of Smiley's book.

Williamson's "Middle Ages" quote appears in Roderick Bailey's *The Wildest Province*, p. 59. The information on the Leskovik raid comes from Naar's unpublished memoir, chapter 11. The LNC "never relaxes" quote comes from an SOE report on 1943 clandestine activities in central and southern Albania, p. 2.

Duffy's heroics during the Shtylle raid are described in a June 21, 1944, SOE memorandum in his personnel file urging that he be considered for a promotion and medal commendation, available at the British National Archives.

The Naar background comes from e-mail, telephone, and in-person interviews, as well as from his unpublished memoir and from his critique of the manuscript. The exchange with Leake appears in chapter 11, p. 2, of Naar's unpublished memoir.

Abbott's "breeze-thumbtack" quote appears on p. 65. The Burgulla hospital chloroform story appears in *Mediterranean Sweep*, p. 338.

The "Ain't Gonna Grieve" story appears on pp. 68–69 of Abbott's book. Steffa's "We do not take prisoners" quote appears on p. 70 of Abbott's book.

Information on what the rest of the 807th squadron was doing back in Catania comes from Dorothy White Errair's history of the 807th MAES, available at the Legends of the Flight Nurses site.

The story questioning Steffa's loyalty appears in Jens's book, pp. 72–73. The growing apprehension about Steffa is covered in Abbott's book, pp. 67–71.

CHAPTER 6:
SURVIVING THE BLIZZARD ON MOUNT TOMORRIT

The stream bathing story appears in Jens's book, p. 75. The new strategy toward getting the attention of the Brits and Lois McKenzie's assertiveness is covered in Jens's book, pp. 75–78.

There's a slight discrepancy between Jens and Abbott on when "Johnny" departed. Abbott says a few days later; again, I'm inclined to go with his version.

Ann Maness's farmhouse recollection comes from her 1991 interview in the WISMA files, as well as information she provided columnist Maury Maverick at the *San Antonio Express-News* for a May 1, 1988, article entitled "Nurses Unsung Heroes of WWII." The *"infermeria"* exchange comes from p. 2 of Maness's 1991 interview. The names of the Berat family members come from Lineberry's book, pp. 222–23.

The march toward Tomorrit is covered in Jens's book, pp. 79–81, and in Abbott's book, pp. 78–80.

The Eldridge stone story comes from Abbott's book, pp. 87–88. The harrowing Tomorrit climb is covered in Jens's book, pp. 87–92, and in Abbott's book, pp. 87–91. The Dawson slip is covered in Jens's book, pp. 88–89; the Rutkowski collapse in Abbott's book, pp. 88–89; and the Cruise-Jens exchange in Jens's book, p. 88. Abbott's "sands run out" quote appears in his book, p. 90. As mentioned in Lineberry's book, Harold Hayes believes that the group climbed the summit of Mount Ostrovice, not Mount Tomorrit. Jens and Abbott both wrote that it was Tomorrit.

The "sizzle and pop" story appears in Abbott's book, p. 91.

Jens's account of the great news from the British captain Smith appears on pp. 91–92 of her book; Abbott's account also appears on pp. 91–92 of his book.

The facial-hair reference appears in Abbott's book, pp. 93–94. Owen's flirtation with the female guerrilla appears in Abbott's book, pp. 94–95.

The "broken minaret" quote comes from the SOE's summary of Albanian clandestine activities in the SOE files at the British National Archives, as do the statistics on the depth of SOE's armament aid to the LNC.

Descriptions of the Davies raid gone awry appear in the Smiley and Kemp books and on p. 36 of Lucas's *OSS*.

The "war of roads" approach appears in the SOE analysis "Albania." The Tare Shyti background comes from information provided via e-mail by Shyti's grandson Leka Bezhani.

A slight discrepancy exists between Jens and Abbott on when the group pushed off for Lovdar. Jens says November 28; Abbott says on or about November 26. This time, my guess is that Jens was probably correct.

Abbott's description of their initial encounter with the British captain Smith appears on pp. 98–99 of his book, Jens's account on pp. 95–96 of her book.

The story of Allen being tossed into the snow by the mule appears in Abbott's book, pp. 99–100. The story of Ann Kopsco being carried into British headquarters appears in Abbott's book, p. 100.

Lieutenant Dawson's offer to take boot sizes appears in Jens's book, p. 104. The descriptions of the Krushove parachute drops appears in Jens's book, pp. 105–10.

The "American women, sir?" story appears in Abbott's book, pp. 103–4.

The background on Major C. Alan Palmer was provided by Jon Naar and the Huntley & Palmers Web site, www.huntleyandpalmers.com.

Abbott's first impression of Duffy taking charge appears on pp. 105–6 of his book. The background information on Duffy comes from his SOE personnel file, Naar's recollections, and from the references to Duffy in books written by Smiley, Kemp, and Roderick Bailey.

The Victor Smith–Korçë story appears in Jens's book, p. 114, the birthday party in Jens's book, pp. 113–14.

The "bodies have arrived!" story appears in Jens's book, p. 119.

The initial reaction to the word about OSS Captain Lloyd Smith appears in Jens's book, pp. 116–20. Abbott's description of Duffy's martial appearances comes from p. 108 of his book.

Jens's "never questioned" Duffy quote comes from her 1995 Betsy Kuhn interview, p. 15.

Naar's story of Churchill triggering the Mena House Hotel fountain was shared over lunch at Union Station in Washington, D.C., November 23, 2012.

Donovan's letter complaining of SOE's obstructionism was written January 8, 1944, and appears in OSS's files at the National Archives II.

CHAPTER 7:
AVERTING A GERMAN AVALANCHE

The VF/LP sign story appears in Abbott's book, p. 107, as does the description of Albanian donkey control.

The Thrasher machine gun story comes from Abbott's book, pp. 106–7.

The Eldridge illness situation is covered in Jens's book, pp. 122–23. The Lebo-Shumway wedding reception anecdote comes from Abbott's book, p. 109.

The Duffy quote about romance appeared in an AP article datelined Cairo, February 15, 1944; it appeared in the *Chicago Daily Tribune* on February 16, 1944, p. 1. There's no byline on the story and the "Cairo" dateline is confusing, but I suspect it was a follow-up piece from Hal Boyle that, like his larger article about the rescue, was suppressed by censors for more than five weeks.

The Cruise quote on romance comes from an interview he gave Lucas for *Rumpalla*, p. 131.

The Maness recollections again come from her 1991 interview on file at WIMSA and the 1988 column in the *San Antonio Express-News*.

The description of the river crossing appears in Jens's book, p. 129.

The Costomicka story appears in Abbott's book, pp. 109–10, although, unlike Jens and Duffy, Abbott spelled it with a "G." The rumors about an Allied invasion of Albania, including Duffy's "nonsense" rebuke, appear in Abbott's book, p. 112.

The Përmet story appears in Jens's book, p. 128.

Their Mount Nemerska experience appears in Abbott's book, pp. 115–19, including the Kanable-Dawson story, p. 119. Lois McKenzie's misgivings about Dawson were conveyed by her daughter Phyllis in an August 2012 phone call.

Lloyd Smith's difficulties in reaching Albania in early December 1943 are covered in the various OSS reports highlighted in Jens's book and available at National Archives II.

The background information on Lloyd Smith comes from his OSS personnel and medal commendation files, available at the National Archives II.

The H. W. Tilman information was initially provided by Jon Naar. The details of Tilman's mountaineering career come from www.mountaineersbooks.org and his SOE personnel and medal commendation files at the British National Archives.

The party's initial close call in Gjirokastër is covered in Jens's book, pp. 134–35.

The pilots' tense conversations with Duffy over a potential air rescue appear in Abbott's book, p. 121, and again on p. 129, and in Jens's book, pp. 142–43.

The story of Duffy helping Jens onto a mule appears in Abbott's book, p. 126. Abbott's "The Huns had us stopped" quote appears on p. 128 of his book.

Lloyd Smith's Vuno automobile story appears in Jens's book, p. 145.

The tense "we'll take responsibility" exchange between Duffy and members of the American party appears in Jens's book, p. 143.

The stories about the shots ringing out in Kalonja and the old woman making the slashing sign across her neck appear in Jens's book, p. 146.

Hasan's boast about blowing up a German staff car appears in Jens's book, pp. 148–49.

The Doksat Christmas stories appear in Jens's book, pp. 152–54, and in Abbott's book, pp. 135–41. The Steffa-Fultz Christmas carol story appears in Jens's book, p. 154.

The Duffy quote about his Irish heritage appears in Jens's book, p. 155.

CHAPTER 8:
THE AIR RESCUE GOES AWRY

"The damper went down" quote appears in Abbott's book, p. 139. The Christmas day menu appears in *Mediterranean Sweep*, p. 239.

Duffy's comments about the nurses' fortitude appear in Jens's book, p. 155.

The Naar quote on "underestimating" the Yanks comes from chapter thirteen of his unpublished memoir, *Time to Tell*. The rest of the information in this section comes from telephone, e-mail, and personal interviews with Naar.

The Germans' surprise occupation of Gjirokastër is covered in Jens's book, pp. 156–58, and in Abbott's book, pp. 141–43.

Elna Schwant's lament about the radio appears in p. 158 of Jens's book.

Naar's recollection of what the armada looked like in Bari appears in chapter thirteen of his unpublished memoir.

The account of the attempted air rescue appears in Jens's book, pp. 162–67, and in Abbott's book, pp. 144–49.

Thrasher's "no broken bones" exchange with Dawson appears on p. 144 of Abbott's book. The "daring the Jerries" to open up quote comes from Abbott's book, p. 146.

Jens's recollection that she could practically "touch" the P-38s comes from the Kuhn 1995 interview, p. 17. Her "beautifully precise formation" description appears in her book, pp. 164–65.

The Adams-Abbott exchange appears on p. 148 of Abbott's book. The frantic race toward the airfield is covered in pp. 146–47 of Abbott's book.

The air armada's success in attacking the German truck formation came from Lloyd Smith's conversation with the escapees on January 7, 1944, and from OSS reports at the National Archives II.

The description of Jens's tears appears on p. 165 of Jens's book.

Duffy's after-action description comes from his SOE files and appears on p. 167 of Jens's book.

Abbott's "walking back on that trail" quote comes from p. 148 of his book.

CHAPTER 9:
CRAWLING AROUND THE ENEMY

The description of how they kept the enemy under surveillance comes from Abbott's book, pp. 152–54. The "They'll blow us to hell" quote comes from Abbott's book, p. 152. Abbott's recollection of how the group was reduced to crawling on hands and knees appears on p. 154 of his book.

Jens's recollection of the family digging a hole to hide its valuables appears on p. 171 of her book.

Jens's New Year's memories, including Elna Schwant's sadness over her missing brother, comes from pp. 171–72 of Jens's book; Abbott's New Year's memories come from p. 154 of his book.

Lloyd Smith's hiring of six guides is covered in an OSS report highlighted in Jens's book, pp. 175–76, and available at National Archives II.

Lois McKenzie's terse exchange with Duffy appears in Jens's book, p. 173.

Jens's wonderful parley with Duffy over the nurses' menstrual cycles appears on pp. 173–74 of her book.

Duffy's report on the people of Saraghinishte appears in his SOE files and on p. 175 of Jens's book.

Baggs's lack of judgment and the group's harrowing ferry crossing appears on pp. 157–59 of Abbott's book.

Pandee's howling appears on pp. 160–61 of Abbott's book; the bonfire story on pp. 161–62. The Golem evening is described in Abbott's book, pp. 162–63.

The Tacina-Duffy exchange is covered in Abbott's book, p. 165.

Duffy bawling out the guide for getting lost in the blizzard is covered in the after-action report in his SOE file, also highlighted in Jens's book, p. 179.

The Eldridge and Dawson mishaps crossing the stream are covered in Abbott's book, pp. 167–68, and in Duffy's after-action report highlighted in Jens's book, pp. 178–81.

CHAPTER 10:
FINAL DASH TO FREEDOM

The initial phyical description of Lloyd Smith appears in Jens's book, pp. 180–83, and in Abbott's book, pp. 166–68. Smith's first exchange with the group is covered in Abbott's book, pp. 167–68, including the Smith-Duffy "why so confident?" exchange.

Lois McKenzie's sardonic "wouldn't that beat all?" quote appears in Jens's book, p. 183.

Lloyd Smith's Terbaci remark also appears in Jens's book, p. 183.

Jens's farewell exchange with Steffa appears on p. 184 of her book. Jens's tearing up of Steffa's note appears on p. 185 of her book.

Steffa's farewell with Abbott appears on p. 170 of his book. Abbott's "Barley Corn Tar" line appears on p. 169 of his book.

Lloyd Smith's dispute with the guide is covered on p. 168 of Abbott's book.

The Sterling Hayden background comes from interviews with Jon Naar and from www.imdb.com/name/nm0001330/bio.

The Bari explosion information comes from the book *Disaster at Bari*, by Glenn B. Infield.

The 807th's response to the Bari tragedy was mentioned in the January 26, 1991, *Leesburg* (Florida) *Daily Commercial*'s article on Nurse Dorothy White Errair and the 807th's history, p. C-1.

Jens's memory of the mules breaking a path in the deep snow appears on p. 188 of her book. Her recollection of being served sugar in her tea appears on pp. 189–90.

Jens's memories of the remarkable truck ride that night appear in her book, pp. 190–93; Abbott's appears in his book, pp. 170–73. Paula Kanable's "elephants" exchange is described in Jens's book, p. 192.

Jim Cruise's exultation appears on p. 173 of Abbott's book. Jens's "we made it" line appears on p. 194 of her book.

Abbott's account of reaching Seaview and climbing aboard the *Yankee* appear on pp. 173–76 of his book; Jens's account of the rescue's final moments appears on pp. 196–98 of her book.

Naar's observation about the U.S. emphasis on public relations comes from his unpublished memoir, as does his recollection of greeting Duffy, Bell, and Williamson. A February 2013 e-mail from Naar described Donovan's greeting of Duffy. The "characteristic understatement" description was also a suggestion from Naar.

Jens's exchange with the G-2 intelligence officer appears on p. 199 of her book.

Hayes's memory of signing four separate confidentiality documents appears in his 1991 interview in the WIMSA files.

The Hal Boyle background information comes from my *Assignment to Hell.*

Jens's postrescue experiences are covered in pp. 211–13 of her book, including her second C-47 crash-landing, this time in Spirit Lake, Iowa. Abbott's postrescue experiences appear in pp. 176–77, including his incredible encounter with the B-25 pilot.

CHAPTER 11:
RESCUING THE MISSING THREE

The OSS's naming of "Champ" and "Underdone" is documented in the OSS files at the National Archives II. The "experience difficulty" quote and other information about Major Smith and Underdone comes from an OSS memo dated January 1944.

The Victor Smith–Alan Palmer rescue attempt is documented in the SOE and OSS after-action reports, some of which are spotlighted in Jens's book, pp. 203–9, and Lucas's *OSS*, pp. 52–53.

The Tare Shyti information was provided by Leka Bezhani, his grandson, and is also described in Ann Maness's 1991 recollections on file at WIMSA, but sans specific references to Tare, since she, Lytle, and Porter never knew his real name.

The Hodo-Kendall-Quayle background is covered in Lucas's *OSS*, p. 52. The Smith-Cooky maneuvering appears in Smith's March 29, 1944, after-action report in the OSS files, National Archives II.

Maness's "nice to get out" quote is from her 1991 interview on file at WIMSA, as is her recollection that the nurses were told to keep their eyes cast toward the ground, as well as her memory of the close calls at German and BK checkpoints.

Smith's March 29, 1944, report in the OSS files is the source of most of the information on the final hours of the Maness-Lytle-Porter escape. Lucas's *OSS* also has an abbreviated account.

Jens's "now complete" line appears on page 209 of her book.

EPILOGUE:
NEVER TOO LATE TO SALUTE HEROES

The Bataan-Corregidor nurses story comes from Doris Weatherford's *American Women During World War II: An Encyclopedia*, pp. 239–41.

The Abbott-Owen "Late Arrival" club information comes from the July 14, 1944, issue of *Yank*, the Army weekly, p. 2.

The information about Abbott's post-Albania World War II experience comes from pp. 189–94 of *Out of Albania*, in an epilogue written by his son, Clint, and from information provided in 2012 Clint via e-mails and telephone interviews. The description of how *Out of Albania* evolved also comes from Clint's epilogue and interviews.

Information on the defeat of German forces in Albania and the triumph of the LNC comes mainly from SOE reports, written contemporaneously, on file at the British National Archives. Most have generic headers, such as "History" or "Albania."

Hoxha's punishment of innocuous crimes information comes from Shyti's grandson Leka Bezhani.

Çela being abandoned by Allied intelligence comes from Lucas's *OSS* and from www.academia.edu/2330113/THE_MOST_SECRET_LIST_OF_SOE_AGENTS. The Shyti house arrest information comes from Leka Bezhani's e-mails from fall 2012 through winter 2013.

The *Detroit Free-Press* article on Tacina and Rutkowski and the *Grand Rapids Press* piece on Jens and Abbott both ran in February 1944. The *Big Rapids Pioneer* article on Jens and Abbott ran on February 25, 1944.

The *Mediterranean Sweep* chapter, "Balkan Journey," appears on pp. 231–43. Lee Whitson's recollection of her mother's misgivings about the pilot came in a December 27, 2012, telephone conversation.

The information about what happened to the SOE operatives comes from conversations with Naar, research conducted by Cameron Smith Howard on Ancestry.com and other sites, and Roderick Bailey's *The Wildest Province*, pp. 322–24.

The Smiley-Philby information comes principally from Naar and "Albania, 1949–1958," available at http://www.globalsecurity.org/intell/ops/albania.htm.

Leake's praise of Duffy came in an SOE memorandum dated March 22, 1944. Much of the rest of the postwar information on Duffy came from Harold Brough's *Liverpool Daily Post* article, February 28, 1995, p. 18.

Jens's memoir, *Albanian Escape: The True Story of U.S. Army Nurses Behind Enemy Lines*, was an "as-told-to" book, coauthored by U.S. wartime nursing historians Evelyn M. Monahan and Rosemary L. Neidel.

The information on Jens's medal commendations comes from Weatherford, pp. 239–41.

Again, the insights about Jean Rutkowski come from conversations and e-mails with her daughter, Lee Whitson.

Harold Hayes's 1961 letter to Larry Abbott was generously provided by Clint Abbott. The information about the fortieth reunion comes from an AP article that appeared in the *Columbus* (Ohio) *Dispatch*, August 31, 1983, and from personal notes now part of the Legends of the Flight Nurses site.

Jens's personal postwar information comes from pp. 211–13 of *Albanian Escape* and from her 2010 memorial service materials, now part of the WIMSA files.

Jens's long quote about Duffy appeared in the *Liverpool Daily Post* article, February 28, 1995.

The information on the Jens-Lucas 1995 trip to Albania appears in Lucas's *Rumpalla*, pp. 137–41.

The personal information on Jim Cruise was in the obituary that appeared in the *Brockton* (Massachusetts) *Enterprise*, July 17, 2010.

The *Newaygo County Times* piece on the Jens-Elna presentation ran on August 15, 2001. The information on the fate of Elna Schwant's brother appears in online information about WWII combat deaths from South Dakota, www.archives.gov/research/arc/ww2/navy-casualties/south-dakota.html.

The prayer was featured in Jens's memorial service materials, provided to WIMSA by her daughter, Karen Mangerich Curtis.

The postwar lives of the nurses were researched by Cameron Smith Howard on various databases, principally Ancestry.com. The information on Dick Lebo's postwar life, including his rebuff of the *Harrisburg Patriot-News*, comes from December 2012–January 2013 e-mails written by Gayle Lebo Yost, his daughter, who also generously provided a copy of the letter she wrote to the newspaper about her dad's World War II service.

The information on Lois Watson McKenzie's postwar life was provided by her daughter Phyllis in phone calls and e-mail notes and referenced in Lois's autobiographical papers.

The "micromanagement" thought comes from a suggestion by Jon Naar via e-mail, March 2013.

The Wouk quote comes from his novel *Inside, Outside* (paperback edition), p. 34.

INDEX